ESSENTIALS OF
Cardiopulmonary
Exercise Testing

Jonathan N. Myers, PhD
Palo Alto Veterans Affairs Medical Center
and
Stanford University

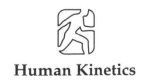

Human Kinetics

Library of Congress Cataloging-in-Publication Data

Myers, Jonathan, 1957-
    Essentials of cardiopulmonary exercise testing / Jonathan N. Myers.
      p.   cm.
    Includes bibliographical references and index.
    ISBN 0-87322-636-4
    1. Exercise tests.   2. Heart function tests.   3. Pulmonary
function tests.   4. Cardiopulmonary system--Diseases--Diagnosis.
I. Title.
    [DNLM: 1. Exercise Test.   2. Respiratory Airflow.   3. Respiratory
Transport.   4. Exercise Tolerance.   WG 141.5.F9 M966E   1996]
RC683.5.E94M94   1996
616.1'20754--dc20
DNLM/DLC
for Library of Congress   96-1015
                                                  CIP

ISBN: 0-87322-636-4

Acquisitions Editor: Richard A. Washburn, PhD; **Developmental Editor**: Ann Brodsky; **Assistant Editor**: Julie Marx Ohnemus; **Editorial Assistants**: Amy Carnes and Coree Schutter; **Copyeditor**: Elaine Otto; **Proofreader**: Karen Bojda; **Typesetter and Layout Artist**: Sandra Meier; **Text Designer**: Judy Henderson; **Pasteup Artist**: Tara Welsch; **Cover Designer**: Jack Davis; **Illustrator**: Tim Offenstein; **Printer**: Braun-Brumfield

Printed in the United States of America

10 9 8 7 6 5 4 3 2 1

Human Kinetics
Web site: http://www.humankinetics.com

United States: Human Kinetics, P.O. Box 5076, Champaign, IL 61825-5076
1-800-747-4457
e-mail: humank@hkusa.com

Canada: Human Kinetics, Box 24040, Windsor, ON N8Y 4Y9
1-800-465-7301 (in Canada only)
e-mail: humank@hkcanada.com

Europe: Human Kinetics, P.O. Box IW14, Leeds LS16 6TR, United Kingdom
(44) 1132 781708
e-mail: humank@hkeurope.com

Australia: Human Kinetics, 57A Price Avenue, Lower Mitcham, South Australia 5062
(08) 277 1555
e-mail: humank@hkaustralia.com

New Zealand: Human Kinetics, P.O. Box 105-231, Auckland 1
(09) 523 3462
e-mail: humank@hknewz.com

CONTENTS

PREFACE

With exercise testing now involving computers, echocardiography, nuclear techniques, pharmacological stress, ventilatory gas exchange analysis, and other applications, it hardly seems adequate to simply write about "exercise testing." So why this book?

Obviously, cardiopulmonary exercise testing has been an area of interest to me for many years. Although an abundance of literature is now available about standard exercise electrocardiography, echo and nuclear techniques, and the roles these play in the assessment of patients with cardiopulmonary disease, such is not the case with gas exchange techniques, an area that remains unfamiliar to many.

The use of gas exchange techniques has expanded in the last two decades. This increase has paralleled an expansion in the area of exercise physiology. No longer restricted to elite athletes, all active people want the latest technology to help them improve performance. More than ever before, gas exchange techniques are used for research, routine testing, and multicenter studies in clinical settings. Though there have been many efforts to predict exercise tolerance or to develop surrogate measures, no measurement of exercise capacity is as precise or as reproducible as directly measured oxygen uptake. Combined with clinical and electrocardiographic data, standard pulmonary function tests, and other exercise data, there is no procedure with as high a yield of clinically useful information.

My recognition of the need for such a text on cardiopulmonary exercise testing grew from interacting with students, nurses, and physicians-in-training through our laboratory and from devoting significant time to teaching the basics of exercise testing and gas exchange techniques. Whereas a cardiology or pulmonary fellow tends to be highly skilled in other areas of patient management, he or she often disregards or misunderstands the interpretation of gas exchange data from an exercise test. Inquiry rarely extends beyond "What was the MET level?" Rarely is there further review of the cardiopulmonary responses or any consideration of whether the MET level was measured directly or predicted from the work rate.

After participating in many multicenter exercise trials employing gas exchange data, I began to appreciate the difficulties of achieving quality control and consistency. There seemed to be as many different methods employed as data collection sites. Many problems involved a lack of basic understanding of gas exchange technology. Thus, I thought a practical reference was needed that technicians, nurses, and other individuals could consult before initiating or performing ongoing studies in a cardiopulmonary exercise testing laboratory.

This book was designed to assist readers who wish to use exercise testing in clinical and research capacities and to gain an appreciation for the measurement, calculation, and application of gas exchange techniques obtained during exercise. An additional aim was to provide a resource for understanding the physiology of cardiopulmonary responses to exercise and basic methods of exercise testing. Thus, in addition to a resource for the clinician, the text can be a useful supplement to a course in exercise or sport science, particularly for anyone preparing for the American College of Sports Medicine certification examinations.

Chapter 1 presents an overview of basic exercise physiology and cardiopulmonary responses to exercise. Chapter 2 focuses on basic exercise testing methodology. (Implicit in the proper application and interpretation of gas exchange techniques is a good understanding of both of these areas.) The next three chapters concentrate specifically on ventilatory gas exchange methods and applications. Chapter 3 discusses instrumentation for measuring gas exchange responses, the many calculations involved, and the underappreciated area of quality control. Chapter 4 reviews the information obtained from gas exchange techniques and discusses its significance. Chapter 5 applies this information to different cardiovascular and pulmonary disorders.

Chapter 6 provides a critique and overview of the literature related to normal (reference) values for exercise capacity. Finally, chapter 7 describes one of the more specialized applications of exercise testing—methods and interpretation of invasive hemodynamic measurements.

You will find the many acronyms associated with these techniques defined in a list of scientific abbreviations and a glossary. These key terms found in the glossary are also highlighted in bold in the text. Appendix A contains equations for predicting oxygen uptake from treadmill and cycle ergometry, along with some examples. Major manufacturers of gas exchange equipment, treadmills, cycle ergometers, ECG systems, and related equipment, along with various related journals and organizations, are listed in appendix B.

This book conveys how exercise testing with gas exchange techniques can be used in clinical and research settings. My intention has been to make the book practical and easily understandable. It is not by any means an exhaustive work, nor is it intended to be, but it is an outgrowth of more than a decade of studies performed in the Cardiovascular Research Laboratories at the Long Beach and Palo Alto Veterans Administration Medical Centers. Many faculty, physicians, visiting cardiologists, cardiology fellows, graduate students, medical students, and nurses have contributed to these studies. Although these individuals are too numerous to mention individually, I've developed knowledge, friendships, and inspiration from all of them, and their contributions pervade the pages of this book.

ACKNOWLEDGMENTS

I wish to gratefully acknowledge Victor Froelicher, MD, for continuing to provide the opportunity and privilege to make a living writing and doing research, and to Eddie Atwood, MD, for all the interest and support over the years. A special thanks to Jill Grumet and Bob Eastlack for their help with the figures, to Bill Herbert, PhD, and Mike Sullivan, MD, for reviewing the manuscript, and particularly to Lesley Anderson for repeatedly but graciously typing the drafts on another of my endeavors.

CREDITS

Figure 1.1 Reprinted, by permission, from VF Froelicher, 1975, "Prediction of maximal oxygen consumption: Comparison of the Bruce and Balke treadmill protocols," *Chest* 68: 333.

Figure 1.2 Reprinted, by permission, from J Myers, 1994, "The physiology behind exercise testing," *Primary Care* 21 (3): 417.

Figure 1.3 Reproduced with permission, from J Myers and VF Froelicher. "Hemodynamic determinants of exercise capacity in chronic heart failure," *Annals of Internal Medicine.* 1991; 115: 378.

Figure 1.4 Reprinted with permission from the American College of Cardiology (*Journal of the American College of Cardiology*, 1993, 22, 177).

Figure 1.5 Reprinted, by permission, from J Myers et al., 1993, "Ventilatory mechanisms of exercise intolerance in chronic heart failure," *American Heart Journal* 124: 711.

Figure 2.2 Reprinted, by permission, from J Myers et al., 1992, "Individualized ramp treadmill: Observations on a new protocol," *Chest* 101: 1340.

Figure 2.3 Reprinted, by permission, from VF Froelicher et al., 1993, *Exercise and the Heart*, 3d ed. (St. Louis: Mosby-Year Book Publishers), 22.

Table 2.3 Reprinted, by permission, from VF Froelicher et al., 1993, *Exercise and the Heart*, 3d ed. (St. Louis: Mosby-Year Book Publishers), 65.

Figure 2.4 Reprinted, by permission, from G Borg, 1985, *An Introduction to Borg's RPE Scale* (Ithaca, NY: Mouvement Publications), 7.

Table 2.4 Reprinted, by permission, from American College of Sports Medicine, 1995, *ACSM Guidelines for Exercise Testing and Prescription*, 5th ed. (Baltimore: Lea & Febiger), 97.

Figure 2.5 Reprinted, by permission, from J Myers et al., 1994, "Increase in blood lactate during ramp exercise: Comparison of continuous versus threshold models," *Medicine and Science in Sport and Exercise* 26: 1413-1419.

Figure 3.7 Reprinted, by permission, from J Myers et al., 1990, "Effect of sampling on variability and plateau in oxygen uptake," *Journal of Applied Physiology* 68: 405.

Figure 4.4 Reprinted, by permission, from VF Froelicher et al., 1993, *Exercise and the Heart*, 3d ed. (St. Louis: Mosby-Year Book Publishers), 40.

Figure 4.5 Reprinted, by permission, from J Myers et al., 1994, "Perception of chest pain during exercise: Testing in patients with coronary artery disease," *Medicine and Science in Sport and Exercise* 26: 1084.

Figure 4.6 Reprinted with permission from the American College of Cardiology (*Journal of the American College of Cardiology*, 1991, 17, 1340).

Figure 4.8 Reprinted, by permission, from J Myers et al., 1989, "Can maximal cardiopulmonary capacity be recognized by a plateau in oxygen uptake?" *Chest* 96: 1314.

Figure 4.9 Reprinted, by permission, from J Myers et al., 1989, "Can maximal cardiopulmonary capacity be recognized by a plateau in oxygen uptake?" *Chest* 96: 1314.

Figure 5.3 Reprinted, by permission, from J Myers et al., 1992, "Ventilatory mechanisms of exercise intolerance in chronic heart failure," *American Heart Journal* 124: 711.

Figure 5.4 Reprinted, by permission, from J Myers et al., 1992, "Ventilatory mechanisms of exercise intolerance in chronic heart failure," *American Heart Journal* 124: 714.

Figure 5.5 Reprinted, by permission, from J Myers et al., 1992, "Ventilatory mechanisms of exercise intolerance in chronic heart failure," *American Heart Journal* 124: 715.

Figure 5.6 Reprinted, by permission, from JE Atwood et al., 1989, "The effect of cardioversion on maximal exercise capacity in patients with chronic atrial fibrillation," *American Heart Journal* 118: 916.

Figure 5.7 Reproduced with permission, from DG Benditt et al., 1987, "Single-chamber cardiac pacing with activity-initiated chronotropic response: Evaluation by cardiopulmonary exercise testing," *Circulation* 75: 190. Copyright 1987 American Heart Association.

Figure 6.1 Reprinted, by permission, from VF Froelicher et al., 1975, "Prediction of maximal oxygen consumption: Comparison of the Bruce and Balke treadmill protocols," *Chest* 68: 334.

Figure 6.2 Reprinted, by permission, from RA Bruce, F Kusumi, and D Hosmer, 1973, "Maximal oxygen uptake and nomographic assessment of functional aerobic impairment in cardiovascular disease," *American Heart Journal* 85: 548.

Figure 6.3 Reprinted with permission from the American College of Cardiology (*Journal of the American College of Cardiology*, 1993, 22, 177).

Figure 6.4 Reprinted with permission from the American College of Cardiology (*Journal of the American College of Cardiology*, 1993, 22, 177).

Figure 6.5 Reprinted with permission from the American College of Cardiology (*Journal of the American College of Cardiology*, 1993, 22, 179).

Figure 6.6 Reprinted with permission from the American College of Cardiology (*Journal of the American College of Cardiology*, 1993, 22, 179).

Figure 7.1 Reprinted, by permission, from MJ Kern, U Deligonul, and C Gudipati, 1991, Hemodynamic and ECG data. In *The Cardiac Catheterization Handbook*, edited by MJ Kern (St. Louis: Mosby-Year Book, Inc.), 103.

INTRODUCTION

> If, then, life is an action of the soul and seems to be greatly aided
> by respiration, how long are we likely to be ignorant of the way in
> which respiration is useful?
>
> Galen of Pergamum

Though the Greek physician Galen (ca. 130-201 A.D.) lacked the benefits of a microprocessor-facilitated test report on his desk when making these observations, he may have been the first to suggest the importance of quantifying respiration accurately. Today we better appreciate that information derived from the volume and pattern of respiration during exercise, measured in a controlled setting, profoundly affects the management of patients with cardiopulmonary disease as well as athletes wishing to maximize physical performance. The procedure used to obtain this information has come to be known as the *cardiopulmonary exercise test*.

Years ago, exercise testing was relatively crude. For example, in the 1920s some of the earliest recordings of ST-segment depression were actually made by having patients perform sit-ups. Exercise testing in the 1930s and 1940s usually meant stepping up and down on a bench for a specified period, during or after which a one-channel recording of the electrocardiogram was obtained. In a survey of exercise testing published in 1971, 45% of laboratories in the United States were using a step procedure for their standard exercise tests. By 1980 a survey of North American laboratories showed this number had dropped to 10-12%. In a survey on methods of exercise testing in the United States and Europe that we conducted in 1995, step tests were virtually nonexistent, having been replaced by microprocessor-controlled treadmills and cycle ergometers.

Not surprisingly, exercise testing today is more sophisticated, is used more widely, and encompasses a wider range of subspecialties, including cardiology, pulmonology, and nuclear medicine. No longer limited to the cardiologist's office, more than 50% of exercise testing today is performed by family practitioners and internists, according to the American College of Physicians. Many cardiologists have encouraged this change, with the primary care provider appropriately serving as gatekeeper to subspecialists.

Use of the exercise test has expanded considerably. It is perhaps the single most important noninvasive procedure used in the management of patients with cardiopulmonary disease. Despite many advances in other technologies related to the detection and management of cardiopulmonary disease, the exercise test continues to be recognized as the most useful first-choice modality in the initial assessment of these patients. In this role, it serves as the major screening test in limiting the use of more expensive and invasive procedures to the most appropriate patients. It remains the most widely used tool in the evaluation of pharmacological therapy and other interventions. In cardiac and pulmonary rehabilitation the exercise test is the cornerstone on which to base the exercise prescription and the primary method by which to measure the efficacy of training. Exercise capacity determined from an exercise test is increasingly recognized as among the most useful clinical measures.

Interestingly, many studies published in the last decade that compare clinical, exercise, and angiographic variables have consistently demonstrated that exercise capacity is the most important variable in risk stratification. To the disappointment of angiographers and surgeons, exercise capacity has been shown to outperform invasive and other noninvasive markers of cardiac performance, including central hemodynamic pressures, markers of ischemia, and other clinically relevant information. Given the results of these studies and the recent shift in health-care policy from process compliance to outcome measures, it stands to reason that exercise capacity should be measured as precisely as possible. The only truly precise measure of exercise capacity comes from gas exchange techniques.

Along with the many expanded applications of the exercise test has come an increase in the use of ventilatory gas exchange techniques, which can

- more accurately quantify exercise capacity,
- evaluate the severity of disease,
- quantify interventions,
- help establish the cause of exertional intolerance,
- establish a foundation for exercise prescription in both health and disease, and
- help determine prognosis.

Despite a major growth in the use of gas exchange techniques during exercise testing, some misinformation nevertheless exists. Thus, it has been a goal of mine for some time to write a work that would better prepare readers not only to obtain and apply this information but also to understand what constitutes misinformation.

Outside the clinical setting, gas exchange technology plays a similarly important, although different, role. Clearly, if a healthy individual wishes to better understand his capabilities or an athlete wishes to determine her cardiopulmonary limits, no other test will provide this information. The classic studies in some of the early exercise laboratories, such as those at Harvard and the University of Minnesota in the 1920s and 1930s, used crude gas exchange methods to evaluate the limits of performance. Some of the observations D.B. Dill, A.V. Hill, Ancel Keys, and others made about the physiological effects of altitude, energy metabolism, oxygen transport, running economy, and predicting endurance performance remain an accepted part of exercise science today. Although the emphasis so often is on the extremes of the spectrum (i.e., patients with severe heart or lung disease or elite athletes), the cardiopulmonary exercise test has been an important medium to better understand the middle—basic human physiology and the mechanisms of a wide variety of diseases. Cardiopulmonary exercise testing has played an integral role in our understanding of nutrition, metabolism, diabetes, rehabilitation from injuries, cardiac and pulmonary rehabilitation, over-training, high altitude physiology, aging, disability, heat illness, and many other areas.

Active people today may simply want to know their "$\dot{V}O_2$max," but exercise testing actually has a variety of applications in sports medicine, including optimizing training and screening cardiac abnormalities. The cardiopulmonary exercise test has formed the basis of literally thousands of research studies on human performance. Whereas cardiac abnormalities in athletic individuals are quite common, serious events are extremely rare. It is no longer considered financially feasible or medically useful to screen apparently healthy, asymptomatic individuals of any age. More often than not, "abnormal" cardiac findings on the ECG, echocardiogram, or cardiac exam in such individuals are variants of normal. Nevertheless, virtually every person who has a serious *event* (i.e., a heart attack or death) during exercise has a serious *disease*—usually of the heart—that adequately explains the event. Such presentations as exercise-induced syncope, exercise-induced asthma, and uncertain chest pain require a complete cardiac workup, and cardiopulmonary exercise testing is the cornerstone of that workup.

Substantial gains have been made in the 1980s and 1990s in technology related to cardiopulmonary exercise testing. Computer-assisted data collection, calibration, and data summary routines were novel concepts when I performed my first exercise tests. Much of the data collection and many of the measurements were performed manually, and cumbersome calculations were made after the test was completed. Much laboratory space was taken up by the gas exchange equipment (including gas analyzers, volume meters, and weather balloons) and devoted to the ECG system. Today this equipment is commonly combined into single, compact units. Intense competition exists between manufacturers to develop systems that are even smaller, more automated, and less expensive, and with greater interest in this technology there are more manufacturers than ever before. This competition can result only in even greater application of the technique.

The study of human physiology is most interesting in the context of the demands of physical stress. Physical performance is an outcome measure that pervades our lives, from the patient disabled by disease to the athlete striving to discover his genetic and physiological limits. The process of measuring these limits of human performance opens a fascinating window into human physiology. Whether using this book as a guide for initiating a cardiopulmonary exercise laboratory, as an additional resource for the more experienced user, or as a supplement for your studies in exercise or sport science, I hope it also serves to further your interest in an important and useful area of science.

CHAPTER 1

CARDIOPULMONARY RESPONSES TO EXERCISE

*E*xercise greatly increases the rate at which oxygen is consumed and carbon dioxide is produced in the muscle. The capacity of the heart and lungs to respond to the stress of exercise is often a measure of their physiological health. This has made the progressive exercise test a well-established and useful tool in clinical medicine. "Cardiopulmonary" exercise suggests that the heart, circulatory system, and lungs function as an integrated unit that takes in, delivers, and exchanges oxygen and carbon dioxide, providing energy and permitting the individual to perform work. Implicit within the term "cardiopulmonary exercise test" is the application of gas exchange technology, in which ventilation into and out of the lungs and the exchange of oxygen and carbon dioxide in the tissues is measured directly.

Why is the direct measurement of gas exchange responses to exercise important? Gas exchange responses permit the user to study the cardiovascular and pulmonary systems simultaneously and to observe directly the pathophysiology of disease states that affect them. The cardiovascular and pulmonary systems are inseparable: placing demands on one without placing equal demands on the other is not possible. Diseases of the heart can cause abnormalities in pulmonary gas exchange, and pulmonary disease can underlie abnormal cardiac responses to exercise. Moreover, gas exchange techniques add precision to the measurement of work. This can be appreciated by reviewing the limitations of predicting **oxygen uptake** and by comparing the reproducibility of measured oxygen uptake with the more common clinical measure of work, exercise time. Proper application of gas exchange technology to the exercise test requires a basic understanding of cardiopulmonary responses to exercise, including basic concepts concerning the measurement of work, the advantages of gas exchange techniques, clinical applications, equipment, and the importance of calibration and quality control. In the following pages, each of these issues will be discussed. This chapter provides an overview of exercise physiology, with the focus on cardiovascular and pulmonary adaptations to acute exercise. The myriad factors that affect the physiologic response to exercise are reviewed, including the type of exercise, age, gender, and environment. Before discussing these cardiopulmonary responses, however, we will review some basic concepts regarding work.

CONCEPTS OF MEASURING AND ESTIMATING WORK

Exercise scientists are frequently concerned with the measurement of **work**. Literally thousands of articles have been published regarding how much work an individual can do, how long work can be sustained and at what intensity, how work can be predicted, and how each of these factors is related to endurance performance or cardiopulmonary function. The ability to measure work has considerable impact on defining the limits of athletic performance as well as the functional capabilities of the patient with cardiovascular disease. The exercise test is a convenient tool with the primary purpose of quantifying the limits of work under controlled conditions.

The many ways that work is expressed have led to some confusion. To help understand this, it is useful to define the basic units of work in metric terms. These include length (in meters), time (in seconds), and mass (in kilograms). Work is defined as force moving through a given distance ($W = F \times D$). **Force** is equal to mass times **acceleration** ($F = M \times A$). Any weight, for example, is a force that is undergoing the acceleration of gravity. A great deal of any work performed involves overcoming the resistance provided by gravity.*

---

*The term ''work'' should not be used synonymously with muscular ''exercise.'' Physiological work (muscle contraction) can occur when no mechanical work (movement) occurs according to physical laws, such as when an isometric contraction is performed.

The basic unit of force is the **newton (N)**. It is the force that, when applied to a 1-kg mass, gives it an acceleration of one meter $\times$ sec^{-2}. Let us return to our original equation for work: W = F (in newtons) $\times$ D (in meters) = Nm. One Nm (newton meter) is equal to one **joule (J)**, which is another common unit of work. Because work is nearly always expressed per unit time (i.e., as a rate), an additional unit that becomes important is **power**, the rate at which work is performed. The body's **metabolic equivalent (MET)** of power is energy. Therefore, it is easy to think of work as anything with weight moving at some rate across time (which is often analogous to distance). These and other useful relationships concerning work are presented in Table 1.1. The common biological measure of total body work is the oxygen uptake, which is usually expressed as a rate (making it a measure of power) in liters per minute.

An accurate measurement of work requires that it be measured directly, which requires that ventilation be quantified precisely and that the concentration of expired oxygen and carbon dioxide be analyzed. (This is covered in more detail in chapter 3.) The direct measurement in oxygen uptake is often not available clinically. It is frequently argued whether the additional and more accurate information gained from exercise testing using gas exchange techniques justifies the added expense, time, and discomfort to the patient. Unfortunately, this question cannot be answered simply yes or no. The answer depends on the purpose of

Table 1.1   Definitions and Useful Relationships Concerning Work

EXPRESSIONS OF WORK:

   Work (W) = Force $\times$ Distance

   Power (P) = Work/Time

   1 kilocaloric (Kcal) = 4.2 kilojoule (kJ)

   1 liter O_2 = 5 Kcal

   1 kg/m = 1.8 ml O_2

EXPRESSIONS OF POWER OR FORCE:

   Power (P) = Work/Time

   Force (F) = Mass $\times$ Acceleration

   Newton meter (Nm) = 1 joule (J)

   1 MET = resting metabolic rate = 3.5 ml/kg/min

   1 MET = 1.0 mph walking on flat surface (1.6 km/hour)

   1 MET = 1 Kcal/kg/hour

   1 watt = 1 J/sec = 1 Nm/sec

   1 watt = 6.1 kgm/min

   1 kilopond (Kp) = 1 kg mass undergoing acceleration of gravity = 9.8 N

   Newton (N) = 1 kgm/sec^2

the test and who is conducting it. In regard to the first consideration, if the purpose of the test is to evaluate an intervention (for example, for research purposes), the limitations of predicting exercise capacity (outlined below) dictate the use of gas exchange techniques. If the purpose of the test is to increase myocardial oxygen demand to an optimal level while obtaining a general estimate of METs (the common clinical expression of exercise capacity), gas exchange techniques generally would not be as useful. In regard to the second consideration, the absence of a good understanding of gas exchange and basic exercise physiology by physicians will likely always be a limitation to the widespread application of gas exchange technology. Gas exchange analysis requires a degree of expertise by the technician, as proper attention to data collection and calibration are essential. At the same time, clinical application of the data requires that the physician possess a basic understanding of ventilatory gas exchange analysis.

An argument will be made throughout this text that work measured directly via gas exchange techniques is much more useful than that estimated from an external workload on a treadmill or cycle ergometer. The decision whether to predict oxygen uptake from the external workload performed or to measure it directly is not trivial, as it can have considerable influence on precision and the yield of information. It may be useful to review some research in this area to put this issue into perspective.

Predicting Oxygen Uptake

Predicting oxygen uptake from the treadmill or cycle ergometer workload is common clinically, but it can be very misleading. Although the two are directly related, with correlation coefficients ranging between 0.8 and 0.9, there is a wide scatter around the regression line. Figure 1.1 illustrates that the 95% confidence limits for predicting oxygen uptake based on treadmill time range more than 30 ml/kg/min (roughly 8.5 METs). This inaccuracy has been attributed to such factors as

- subject habituation (less variation occurs with treadmill experience);
- fitness (less variation occurs with increased fitness);
- the presence of heart disease (oxygen uptake is overpredicted for diseased individuals);
- handrail holding (the oxygen cost of the work is markedly reduced if the subject is allowed to hold on to the handrails); and
- the exercise protocol (less variation occurs when more gradual, individualized protocols are used).

Thus, if quantifying work with precision is an important objective, such as in research studies, a direct measurement is essential. Equations commonly used for predicting oxygen uptake on a treadmill and cycle ergometer are presented in appendix A.

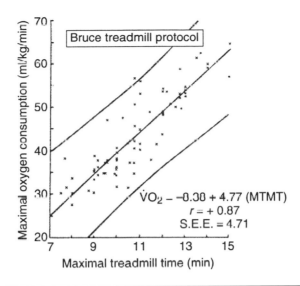

Figure 1.1 Relationship between maximal oxygen uptake and maximal treadmill time among 77 men tested using the Bruce protocol. Outer lines represent the 95% confidence limits. SEE = standard error of the estimate; MTMT = maximal treadmill exercise time. Reprinted from Froelicher 1975.

Numerous studies describe the factors affecting the relationship between measured and predicted oxygen uptake. The wide scatter around the regression line between oxygen uptake and exercise time or workload is well documented yet poorly appreciated. Most pharmaceutical trials, for example, continue to report work in terms of the relatively unreliable measure, exercise time. This is particularly a concern since many studies have shown that the presence of heart disease can greatly increase the error associated with predicting oxygen uptake. Sullivan and McKirnan (1) reported that measured oxygen uptake was 13% lower among patients with coronary disease than among normal subjects for the same treadmill work at higher levels of exercise. Roberts et al. (2) evaluated the relationship between measured and predicted oxygen uptake in a heterogeneous group of patients with heart disease and a group of normals. Measured oxygen uptake was lower at matched work rates throughout exercise among the patients. Moreover, the discrepancy between the two groups became progressively greater as exercise progressed: at higher levels of exercise, differences as large as one MET were observed. This difference between oxygen uptake measured among the patients and that predicted from the workload was even greater: at high levels of exercise, oxygen uptake was overpredicted by roughly 2.5 METs.

The slope of the relationship between measured and predicted oxygen uptake was recently compared among patients with heart disease and age-matched normals on a variety of treadmill and cycle ergometer protocols (3). A slope represents a change in an independent variable (in this case, an increment in treadmill or cycle ergometer work) for a given change in a dependent variable (here measured oxygen uptake). Thus, a slope equal to 1.0 would be observed if the variables changed in direct proportion to one another. This is never the case, however, even among normals. Table 1.2 illustrates that patients with chronic heart failure or coronary disease and those limited by angina on the treadmill have significantly reduced slopes (ranging from 0.51 to 0.53) compared with normals (slope 0.71). The common explanation for the reduced oxygen uptake values at matched work rates is the cardiopulmonary system's inability to adapt to the demands of the work. Not surprisingly, patients with chronic heart failure are particularly known to exhibit this response, and the effects of beta-blockade (i.e., reduced heart rate, cardiac output, and oxygen uptake) on this response must also be considered when using workload to predict oxygen uptake (4,5).

The choice of exercise protocol is also known to influence the relationship between measured and predicted work. Haskell et al. (6), for example, reported that estimating oxygen uptake among patients with heart disease was valid only if a gradual protocol was used. Using an accelerated protocol, peak $\dot{V}O_2$ was significantly overestimated. Our laboratory recently evaluated differences among six protocols in terms of the relationship between measured and predicted oxygen uptake (3). Three treadmill and three cycle ergometer protocols were compared. The three treadmill protocols used were a gradual (modified Balke), a rapid (standard Bruce), and a moderately incremented test (individualized ramp). The three cycle ergometer protocols were a rapid (50 watts/stage), a gradual (25 watts/stage), and a moderately incremented test (individualized ramp). Among 31 patients with heart disease and 10 normals, the slope of the relationship between measured and predicted oxygen uptake was quantified throughout exercise.

Table 1.3 presents the slopes of these relationships for each protocol. The protocols with the largest increments in work (i.e., Bruce treadmill and 50 watts/

Table 1.2   Slopes in Oxygen Uptake Versus Work Rate for Each Patient Subgroup Performing Each of Six Exercise Protocols

	Coronary artery disease	Angina	Chronic heart failure	Normal
Slope	0.51	0.53	0.53	0.71*
SEE, ml O₂/kg/min	2.6	3.1	2.8	4.2

*$p < 0.001$ versus other groups.

SEE = standard error of the estimate.

If the change in ventilatory oxygen uptake were equal to the change in work rate, the slope would be equal to 1.0.

Data from Myers et al., J Am Coll Cardiol 1991; 17:1334-1342.

Table 1.3   Slopes in Oxygen Uptake Versus Work Rate for 40 Subjects Performing Six Exercise Protocols

	Treadmill			Bicycle		
	Bruce	Balke	Ramp	25 W	50 W	Ramp
Slope	0.62	0.79	0.80	0.69	0.59	0.78
SEE	4.0	3.4	2.5	2.3	2.8	1.7

SEE = standard error of the estimate (ml O_2/kg/min); 25 W = 25 watts/stage; 50 W = 50 watts/stage.

Each slope ≥ 0.78 was significantly different from each slope ≤ 0.69 ($p < 0.05$ except Balke versus 25 W, $p = 0.07$). If the change in ventilatory oxygen uptake were equal to the change in work rate, the slope would be equal to 1.0.

stage cycle ergometer) have slopes that were significantly lower than those with smaller increments in work. This suggests that protocols which increase rapidly or have large increments in work overpredict exercise capacity. In addition, the standard error of the estimate (oxygen uptake, ml/kg/min) was largest for the Bruce test and smallest for the individualized ramp tests, suggesting that the variability in estimating oxygen uptake from workload is greater for rapidly incremented tests versus those that are more gradual and/or individualized.

Reproducibility

An important consideration, particularly when serially testing patients for research protocols such as pharmaceutical trials, is the reliability and reproducibility of the data. This has been one of the most important arguments in favor of the use of gas exchange techniques. The tendency to increase treadmill time with serial testing without an increase in maximal oxygen uptake is well documented. Many large multicenter drug trials in cardiology have shown significant increases in exercise time on placebo treatment that could be attributed only to repeated testing, sometimes concealing any salutary effects of therapy.

Changes in treadmill time with serial testing have even been observed without changes in maximal heart rate or double product (7). Elborn et al. (8) performed three consecutive treadmill tests on separate days in patients with heart failure and reported that the first test underestimated exercise capacity by approximately 20%. Pinsky et al. (9) performed repeated treadmill tests among patients with heart failure until test duration on three consecutive tests varied by less than 60 sec (a common qualification criteria for pharmaceutical trials). This stability criterion was achieved within three tests on only 9 of 30 patients, whereas 13 patients required four or five tests and 8 patients required more than six tests.

Sullivan and associates (10) compared the reproducibility of treadmill time and oxygen uptake among patients with angina tested on three days within a week. Measured oxygen uptake had a higher intraclass correlation coefficient ($r = 0.88$) than treadmill time ($r = 0.70$) across the three exercise tests on different days (Table 1.4). In addition, the 90% confidence intervals for the intraclass correlation coefficients were higher for measured oxygen uptake ($r = 0.76$ to 0.95) than for treadmill time ($r = 0.48$ to 0.86). Thus, gas exchange techniques yield a more reliable, reproducible, and accurate assessment of exercise capacity and cardiopulmonary function than treadmill time or workload achieved. In our view, this technology is essential when using exercise as an efficacy parameter to study interventions.

PHYSIOLOGIC RESPONSES TO EXERCISE

Exercise is the body's most common physiologic stress; it places major demands on the cardiopulmonary system. Maximal exercise can define the limits of performance in a healthy individual or the functional capabilities of the patient with heart disease. The exercise test has therefore been a valuable clinical tool for assessing therapy in patients with various cardiovascular disorders under controlled conditions. Virtually all body systems, including the pulmonary, endocrine, neuromotor, and thermoregulatory, are involved in the homeostatic adjustments required for acute exercise and in the chronic adaptations that occur with physical training. These adaptations allow the body to increase its metabolic rate up to 20 times the resting rate, during which cardiac output may increase as much as 6 times. The magnitude of these adaptations is dependent upon an individual's age, sex, body size, fitness, the type of exercise, and the presence or absence of heart disease. Let us begin with a profile of the physiologic responses to acute exercise with an emphasis on the cardiopulmonary system, followed by an overview of respiratory gas exchange.

Table 1.4   Mean ± SD for Oxygen Uptake and Treadmill Time at Peak Angina-Limited Exercise for 14 Patients

	Day 1	Day 2	Day 3	ICC	90% confidence interval for ICC
Time (sec)	503 ± 72	516 ± 85	526 ± 66	0.70	0.48-0.86
Oxygen uptake (L/min)	1.56 ± 0.29	1.55 ± 0.33	1.56 ± 0.29	0.88	0.76-0.95

ICC = intraclass correlation coefficient.

Acute Cardiopulmonary Response to Exercise

The cardiovascular system responds to acute exercise with a series of adjustments that ensure that

- active muscles receive blood supply appropriate to their metabolic needs,
- heat generated by the muscles is dissipated, and
- blood supply to the brain and heart is maintained.

This requires a major redistribution of cardiac output along with some local metabolic changes. The extent to which basic hemodynamic and metabolic variables change from rest to a moderately high level of exercise is illustrated in Figure 1.2. The volume of blood pumped by the heart is commonly expressed in liters per minute and called the **cardiac output ($\dot{Q}$)**. Cardiac output is determined by the product of heart rate (beats/min) and **stroke volume** (ml/beat), and it is a principal factor governing the delivery and use of oxygen by the working tissues.

The usual measure of the capacity of the body to deliver and use oxygen is the maximal oxygen uptake ($\dot{V}O_2$max). No other measure of work is as encompassing, precise, or reproducible as $\dot{V}O_2$max. Thus, the upper limits of the cardiopulmonary system are historically defined by $\dot{V}O_2$max, which can be expressed by the **Fick principle**:

$$\dot{V}O_2\text{max} = \text{Maximal Cardiac Output} \times$$
$$\text{Maximal Arteriovenous Oxygen Difference}$$

The cardiopulmonary limits ($\dot{V}O_2$max) are therefore defined by a central component (cardiac output), which describes the capacity of the heart to function as a pump, and peripheral factors **(arteriovenous oxygen difference)**, which describe the capacity of the lung to oxygenate the blood delivered to it and the capacity of the working muscle to extract this oxygen from the blood. Figure 1.3 (p. 11) outlines the many factors that affect cardiac output and arteriovenous oxygen difference. Often, an abnormality in one or more of these factors determines the presence and extent of cardiovascular or pulmonary disease.

Oxygen uptake increases linearly with increasing work. Traditionally, oxygen uptake has been termed maximal when it no longer increases with increasing work (i.e., it plateaus). However, the plateau concept has recently fallen into some disfavor because it is frequently not observed in patients with heart disease, it is poorly reproducible, and it depends greatly on how gas exchange data are sampled and the criteria applied (12-14). (This is discussed further in chapter 4.) $\dot{V}O_2$max may reach levels as high as 4-5 L/min in young, fit individuals, commensurate with an increase in the resting metabolic rate of 15 to 20 times. Because $\dot{V}O_2$max is related to body weight, it is commonly adjusted for weight in kilograms; normal values for healthy adults generally range from 25 to 50 ml/kg/min.

Cardiac output must closely match ventilation in the lung to deliver oxygenated blood to the working muscle. $\dot{V}O_2$max can also be expressed by the maximal

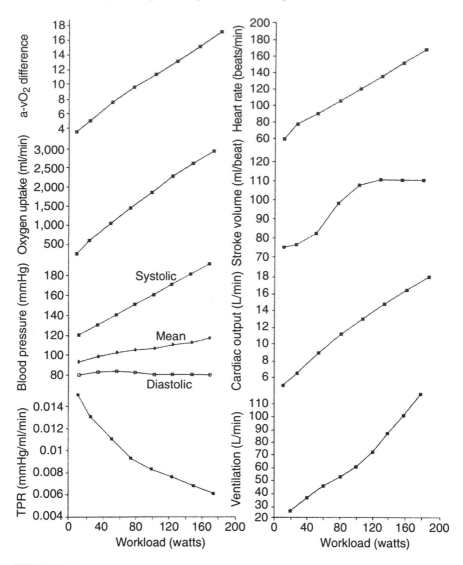

Figure 1.2 Response of basic hemodynamic and metabolic variables from rest to a moderately high level of exercise in the upright position. Reprinted from Myers 1994.

amount of ventilation moving into and out of the lung and the fraction of oxygen in this ventilation extracted by the tissues:

$$\dot{V}O_2 = \dot{V}_E \times (F_IO_2 - F_EO_2),$$

where $\dot{V}_E$ is **minute ventilation** and F_IO_2 and F_EO_2 are the fractional amounts of oxygen in the inspired and expired air, respectively. (The equation above is

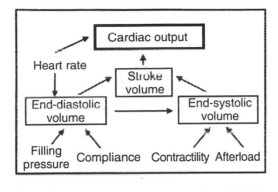

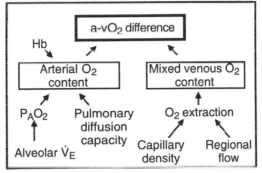

Figure 1.3 Central and peripheral determinants of maximal oxygen uptake. a-vO$_2$ difference = the difference between arterial and venous oxygen; Hb = hemoglobin; $\dot{V}_E$ = minute ventilation; P$_A$O$_2$ = partial pressure of alveolar oxygen. Reprinted from Myers and Froelicher 1991.

oversimplified for the moment as it makes several assumptions; more on this in chapter 3). Thus, the physiologic response to exercise requires the integration of cardiac, pulmonary, and peripheral components. In the following pages, the model illustrated in Figure 1.3 is reviewed in the context of the cardiovascular response to exercise.

Central Factors

Central adaptations to acute exercise refer to those factors which influence the capacity of the heart to receive and eject blood and therefore provide oxygen to the working tissues. These factors include heart rate, stroke volume, filling pressure, ventricular compliance, contractility, afterload, and ventricular volume responses.

Heart Rate

Sympathetic and parasympathetic nervous system influences underlie the cardiovascular system's first response to exercise, an increase in heart rate. Sympathetic outflow increases to the heart and systemic blood vessels and vagal outflow decreases. Of the two major components of cardiac output, heart rate and stroke volume, heart rate is responsible for most of the increase in cardiac output during exercise, particularly at higher levels. Heart rate increases linearly with workload and oxygen uptake. Increases in heart rate occur primarily at the expense of diastolic, not systolic, time. Thus, at very high heart rates, such as might be observed in a patient with atrial fibrillation, diastolic time may be so short as to preclude adequate ventricular filling.

The heart rate response to exercise is influenced by several factors, including (15)

- age,
- type of activity,
- body position,
- fitness,
- the presence of heart disease,
- medications,
- blood volume, and
- environment.

Of these, perhaps the most important is age: a decline in maximal heart rate occurs with increasing age (Figure 1.4). This appears to be due to intrinsic cardiac changes rather than to neural influences. It should be noted that much variability occurs around the regression line between maximal heart rate and age; thus, age-related maximal heart rate is a relatively poor index of maximal effort (15,16).

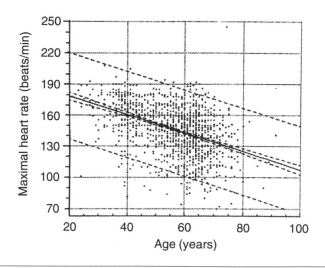

Figure 1.4   The relationship between maximal heart rate and age among 1,388 patients referred for exercise testing for clinical reasons. Inner lines represent the standard error; outer lines represent 95% confidence limits. Reprinted from Morris et al. 1993.

Maximal heart rate is unchanged or may be slightly reduced after a program of training. Resting heart rate is frequently reduced after training, which is due to enhanced parasympathetic tone.

Stroke Volume

The product of stroke volume (the volume of blood ejected per heartbeat) and heart rate determines cardiac output. Stroke volume (SV) is equal to the difference between **end-diastolic** and **end-systolic volume**. Thus, a greater diastolic filling (**preload**) will increase stroke volume. Factors that increase arterial blood pressure will resist ventricular outflow (**afterload**) and result in a reduced stroke volume. During exercise, stroke volume increases to 50% to 60% of maximal capacity, after which increases in cardiac output are caused by further increases in heart rate. The extent to which increases in stroke volume during exercise reflect an increase in end-diastolic volume and/or a decrease in end-systolic volume is not entirely clear, but it appears to depend on ventricular function, body position, and intensity of exercise. In healthy subjects, stroke volume increases at rest and throughout exercise after a period of exercise training. Although this has been argued, evidence suggests that increases in stroke volume after training are due more to increases in preload and possibly local adaptations that reduce peripheral vascular resistance than to increases in myocardial contractility.

In addition to heart rate, end-diastolic volume is determined by two other factors: **filling pressure** and **ventricular compliance**.

Filling Pressure

The most important determinant of ventricular filling is venous pressure. The degree of venous pressure is a direct consequence of venous return. The **Frank Starling mechanism** dictates that, within limits, all blood returned to the heart will be ejected during systole. As the tissues demand greater oxygen during exercise, venous return increases, which increases end-diastolic fiber length (preload), resulting in a more forceful contraction. Venous pressure increases as exercise intensity increases. Over the course of a few beats, cardiac output will equal venous return.

A number of other factors affect venous pressure and therefore filling pressure during exercise. These include blood volume, body position, and the pumping action of the respiratory and skeletal muscles. A greater blood volume increases venous pressure and therefore end-diastolic volume by making more blood available to the heart. Filling pressure is greatest in the supine position because the effects of gravity are negated. In fact, stroke volume generally does not increase from rest to maximal exercise in the supine position. The intermittent mechanical constriction and relaxation of the skeletal muscles during exercise also enhance venous return. Lastly, changes in intrathoracic pressure that occur with breathing during exercise facilitate the return of blood to the heart.

Ventricular Compliance

Compliance is a measure of the capacity of the ventricle to stretch in response to a given volume of blood. Specifically, compliance is defined as the ratio of the change in volume to the change in pressure:

$$\text{Compliance} = \Delta \text{ Volume} / \Delta \text{ Pressure}$$

The diastolic pressure/volume relation is curvilinear; i.e., at high end-diastolic pressures, small changes in volume are accompanied by large changes in pressure. At the upper limits of end-diastolic pressure, ventricular compliance declines, that is, the chamber becomes stiffer as it fills. Because of the difficulty of measuring end-diastolic pressure during exercise, few data are available concerning ventricular compliance during exercise in humans.

End-systolic volume, which will now be addressed, is a function of two factors: **contractility** and afterload.

Contractility

Contractility describes the force of the heart's contraction. Increasing contractility reduces end-systolic volume, which results in a greater stroke volume and thus cardiac output. This is precisely what occurs with exercise in the normal individual: the amount of blood in the ventricle that is ejected with each beat increases, owing to an altered cross-bridge formation. Contractility is commonly quantified by the **ejection fraction**: the percentage of blood ejected from the ventricle during systole measured using radionuclide, echocardiographic, or angiographic techniques. Despite its wide application as an index of myocardial contractility, ejection fraction has repeatedly been shown to correlate poorly with exercise capacity (Figure 1.5) (17-19).

Afterload

Afterload is a measure of the force resisting the ejection of blood by the heart. Increased afterload (or aortic pressure, as is observed with chronic hypertension) results in a reduced ejection fraction and increases in end-diastolic and end-systolic volumes. During dynamic exercise, the force resisting ejection in the periphery **(total peripheral resistance)** is reduced by vasodilation, owing to the effect of local metabolites on the skeletal muscle vasculature. Thus, despite even a fivefold increase in cardiac output among normals during exercise, mean arterial pressure increases only moderately.

Ventricular Volume Response to Exercise

Results of studies evaluating the volume response to exercise have varied greatly. Although the arrival of radionuclide techniques in the 1970s offered promise for the noninvasive assessment of ventricular volumes during exercise, their success

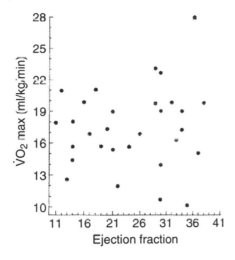

Figure 1.5 The relationship between resting left ventricular ejection fraction and maximal oxygen uptake ($\dot{V}O_2$max) in patients with chronic heart failure ($r = 0.13$, not significant). Reprinted from Myers et al. 1993.

has been only modest. Because of technical limitations, many of these studies have been performed in the supine position. The volume response to exercise appears to depend on the

- presence and type of disease,
- method of measurement (radionuclide or echocardiographic),
- type of exercise (supine versus upright), and
- exercise intensity (submaximal versus maximal).

Much of the disagreement no doubt can be attributed to differences in the exercise level at which measurements were performed. With this in mind, some rough generalizations may be made concerning changes in ventricular volume in response to upright exercise (20-28).

In normal subjects, the response from upright rest to a moderate level of exercise is an increase in both end-diastolic and end-systolic volume, roughly in the order of 15% and 30%, respectively. As exercise progresses to a higher intensity, end-diastolic volume probably does not increase further (27), while end-systolic volume decreases progressively. At peak exercise, end-diastolic volume may even decline while stroke volume is maintained by a progressively decreasing end-systolic volume.

Among several studies that have quantified the volume response to exercise among patients with coronary artery disease in the upright position (21,23,29-31), end-diastolic volume has been reported to increase between 16% and 56%. The increase in end-systolic volume has been reported to range from 16% to 48%. An exception, however, is a study performed by Rerych and associates

(23), who reported a 94% increase in end-systolic volume. Among patients with chronic heart failure, Sullivan et al. (32) reported approximately 20% increases in both end-diastolic and end-systolic volumes from rest to maximal upright exercise. Few data are available in this group in the upright position. A summary of the major studies using upright exercise is presented in Table 1.5 (21-35).

Peripheral Factors

Oxygen extraction by the tissues during exercise reflects the difference between the oxygen content of the arteries (generally 18 to 20 ml O_2/100 ml at rest) and the oxygen content of the veins (generally 13 to 15 ml O_2/100 ml at rest, yielding a resting a-vO_2 difference of 4 to 5 ml O_2/100 ml, approximately 23% extraction). During exercise, this difference widens as the working tissues extract greater amounts of oxygen. Venous oxygen content reaches very low levels, and a-vO_2 difference may be as high as 16 to 18 ml O_2/100 ml with exhaustive exercise (exceeding 85% extraction of oxygen from the blood at $\dot{V}O_2$max). Some oxygenated blood always returns to the heart, as smaller amounts of blood continue to flow through metabolically less active tissues that do not fully extract oxygen. Generally, a-vO_2 difference does not explain differences in $\dot{V}O_2$max among subjects who are relatively homogeneous. That is, a-vO_2 difference is generally considered to widen by a fixed amount during exercise, and differences in $\dot{V}O_2$max have been historically explained by differences in cardiac output. However, many patients with cardiovascular and pulmonary disease exhibit reduced $\dot{V}O_2$max values that can be attributed to a combination of central and peripheral factors.

Determinants of Arterial Oxygen Content

Arterial oxygen content is related to the **partial pressure** of arterial oxygen, which is determined in the lung by **alveolar ventilation** ($\dot{V}_A$) and pulmonary

Table 1.5   Summary of Studies Evaluating Ventricular Volume Responses to Upright Exercise Using Radionuclide or Echocardiographic Techniques

Population	Mean (%) change EDV (range)	Mean (%) change ESV (range)
Normals*	11.0 (−26 to +45)	−24.9 (−65 to +48)
Coronary artery disease**	24.0 (+8 to +56)	41.6 (+16 to +94)
Chronic heart failure***	20.0	20.0

EDV = end-diastolic volume; ESV = end-systolic volume.
*References 21-30, 33.
**References 21, 23, 29-31, 33-35.
***Reference 32.

diffusion capacity and in the blood by **hemoglobin** content. In the absence of pulmonary disease, arterial oxygen content and saturation generally remain similar to resting values throughout exercise, even at very high levels. This is true even among most patients with severe coronary disease or chronic heart failure. Patients with pulmonary disease, however, often neither ventilate the alveoli adequately nor diffuse oxygen from the lung into the blood normally, and a decrease in oxygen saturation during exercise is a hallmark of this disorder. Arterial hemoglobin content is also usually normal throughout exercise. Naturally, a condition such as anemia would reduce the oxygen-carrying capacity of the blood. Conditions that shift the oxyhemoglobin dissociation curve (which reflects the degree of hemoglobin saturation for any given partial pressure of oxygen) leftward, such as reduced 2,3 diphosphoglycerate, PCO_2, or temperature, would also reduce the oxygen-carrying capacity of the blood.

Determinants of Venous Oxygen Content

Venous oxygen content reflects the capacity to extract oxygen from the blood as it flows through the muscle. It is determined by the amount of blood directed to the muscle (regional flow) and capillary density. Muscle blood flow increases in proportion to the increase in work rate and thus the oxygen requirement. The increase in blood flow is brought about not only by the increase in cardiac output but also by a preferential redistribution of the cardiac output to the exercising muscle (Figure 1.6). More than 85% of the total cardiac output may be redistributed to the skeletal muscle at high levels of exercise. A reduction in local vascular resistance facilitates this greater skeletal muscle flow; systemic vascular resistance decreases twofold to threefold during exercise. In turn, locally produced vasodilatory mechanisms and possible neurogenic dilatation caused by higher sympathetic activity mediate the greater skeletal muscle blood flow. A marked increase

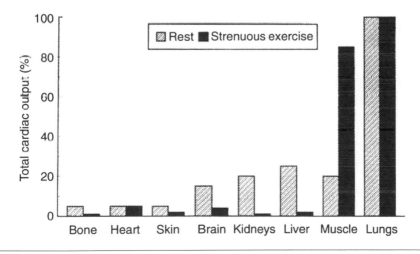

Figure 1.6   Changes in the distribution of cardiac output from rest to strenuous work.

in the number of open capillaries reduces diffusion distances, increases capillary blood volume, and increases mean transit time, facilitating oxygen delivery to the muscle.

In cross-sectional studies, fit individuals have been shown to exhibit a greater skeletal muscle capillary density than sedentary subjects. Advances in histochemical techniques have permitted the demonstration of increases in the number of capillaries and higher capillary to fiber ratios after training (36-38). Many skeletal muscle adaptations to training appear to be reversible with deconditioning (38). In addition, fit subjects may have a greater capacity to redistribute blood flow toward the working muscles and away from nonexercising tissue. Interestingly, one characteristic of the patient with chronic heart failure is an "exaggeration" of the deconditioning response. These patients exhibit a reduced capacity to redistribute blood, a reduced capacity to vasodilate in response to exercise or following ischemia, and a reduced capillary to fiber ratio (18).

Responses of the Pulmonary System

To perform large amounts of work, an individual must take a large amount of air into the lungs. Air moving into and out of the lungs is usually measured in liters per minute, expressed as minute ventilation ($\dot{V}_E$, body temperature and pressure, saturated [**BTPS**]) and can be easily quantified today with automated techniques. Maximal $\dot{V}_E$ is an important component of cardiopulmonary performance. In order for the skeletal muscle to consume oxygen, blood must be delivered to the lungs by the heart, ventilation must match cardiac output in the lungs, and efficient gas exchange must occur. Inefficient ventilation, even in the absence of clinically apparent pulmonary disease, contributes to abnormal exercise responses in certain disease states.

Minute ventilation increases from roughly 8 to 12 L/min at rest to more than 150 L/min at peak exercise in highly fit individuals. Increases in minute ventilation are achieved by increases in both **tidal volume** (V_T, the amount of air inhaled or exhaled) and respiratory rate, with respiratory rate accounting for most of the increase in ventilation at higher levels of exercise. The large increase in pulmonary blood flow during exercise is accompanied by an approximate twofold reduction in pulmonary vascular resistance and a moderate increase in pulmonary artery pressure. A portion of the increased pulmonary flow goes to underperfused areas of the lungs, so that ventilation and perfusion are more equally matched and **ventilatory dead space** (V_D) decreases slightly.

The major factors governing adaptations of the pulmonary system to exercise are gas exchange in the lungs (the transfer of oxygen and carbon dioxide between the lungs and blood) and the physiological determinants of the ventilatory requirement for exercise.

Gas Transfer in the Lungs and Tissues

The exchange of O_2 and CO_2 between the lungs, tissues, and blood occurs by **diffusion**, the passive tendency of a molecule to move from a region of higher to one of lower concentration. The rate of gas diffusion through a tissue is proportional to the tissue surface area (in the lung it is very large, about 50 to 100 m^2) and to the difference in the partial pressure of the gas between the two sides of the capillary. Oxygen, for example, has a partial pressure (PO$_2$) of roughly 100 mmHg in the pulmonary and arterial blood but only 40 mmHg in the skeletal muscle. This large gradient causes O$_2$ to diffuse readily from the arterial blood to the muscle. On the other hand, the difference in partial pressure of CO$_2$ (PCO$_2$) between the venous blood and the pulmonary capillaries is only about 6 mmHg (46 versus 40), but its high solubility causes it to be diffused rapidly from the venous blood to the lung, where it is exhaled. The pressure gradients that facilitate gas transfer in the lung and skeletal muscles are illustrated in Figure 1.7.

Gas transfer in the normal lung is rapid: less than one second is needed to achieve equilibrium between the blood and alveolar gas. Even during heavy exercise, the speed with which the red blood cells pass through the pulmonary capillaries remains about half that at rest. This is possible in part because the pulmonary capillaries can increase the volume of blood contained within them by threefold. This enables the body to maintain an arterial PO$_2$ of nearly 100 mmHg and a PCO$_2$ of 40 mmHg, even with severe exercise.

Determinants of the Ventilatory Requirement for Exercise

The ventilatory requirement for exercise relates primarily to CO$_2$ clearance from the blood and, therefore, CO$_2$ exchange in the lungs. For moderate levels of exercise, arterial **pH** is maintained when arterial PCO$_2$ is maintained. For this to occur, alveolar $\dot{V}_E$ must increase in accordance with the rate at which CO$_2$ is produced. Under these ideal conditions, alveolar PO$_2$ and PCO$_2$ are equal to those

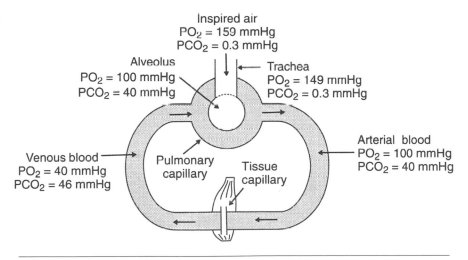

Figure 1.7   Pressure gradients throughout the circulatory system for gas exchange at rest.

in the arterial blood, and pulmonary gas exchange (oxygen uptake, expired CO_2) occurs in accordance with the rate at which the alveoli are ventilated.

In reality, however, some of the ventilated air does not reach the alveoli and participate in gas exchange, and some air reaches nonperfused areas of the lungs. This difference between minute ventilation ($\dot{V}_E$) and air participating in gas exchange is the dead space fraction of $\dot{V}_E$, expressed as a fraction of the tidal volume (V_D/V_T). Thus, the ventilatory requirement for a given amount of work requires knowledge of its three most important determinants and their interaction:

$$\dot{V}_E \text{ (BTPS)} = \frac{863 \ \dot{V}CO_2 \text{ (STPD)}}{P_aCO_2 \ (1 - V_D/V_T)},$$

where BTPS and **STPD** (standard temperature and pressure, dry) are the conventional conditions under which $\dot{V}_E$ and $\dot{V}CO_2$ are expressed, 863 is a correction for these conditions, and P_aCO_2 is the partial pressure of arterial CO_2. (These issues are raised again in chapters 3, 4, and 5.)

FACTORS AFFECTING THE RESPONSE TO EXERCISE

Both hemodynamic responses and maximal values can be greatly influenced by the type of exercise employed. A great deal of research has been performed comparing exercise modes, protocols, static versus dynamic exercise, exercise positions, arm versus leg exercise, and acute versus endurance responses. Each is addressed briefly.

Exercise Mode

It is well established that variations in $\dot{V}O_2$max generally reflect the quantity of muscle mass activated (39,40). Numerous studies have reported 10% to 20% higher values for $\dot{V}O_2$max when exercise is performed on a treadmill compared with cycle ergometers or other exercise modes (3,41,42). Exercise tests using arm ergometry yield peak oxygen uptake values roughly 70% of those achieved on a treadmill or cycle ergometer (43,44). The smaller muscle mass employed using upper arm versus leg work leads to higher blood pressures, higher heart rates, and presumably higher ventricular wall stress and myocardial oxygen demand at matched work intensities (45-47). However, a clear training specificity has been observed in many studies among athletes; higher maximal oxygen uptake values are often achieved among swimmers or cyclists who are tested in the sport in which they are trained (48-51).

Exercise Protocol

The many exercise testing protocols in use have led to some confusion regarding the interpretation of responses to exercise. In general, maximal values for heart rate or oxygen uptake are not markedly different between protocols as long as the same mode is used (3). However, gas exchange dynamics can vary greatly by altering the way work is incremented on a treadmill or cycle ergometer. Several investigators have recently recommended using more gradual, equally incremented, or ramping protocols when testing patients with heart disease (3,42,52-58). Such protocols permit a more accurate estimate of exercise capacity (3,57,58), are more reliable for studying the effects of therapy (52,53,59), and may even be more sensitive for detecting coronary disease (54).

Supine Versus Upright Exercise

Supine exercise has been particularly useful for radionuclide studies or when acquiring hemodynamic measurements during exercise in the catheterization laboratory. However, supine exercise can be awkward, and exercise capacity is considerably lower than when performed in the upright position. In addition, hemodynamic responses to exercise differ considerably. Because gravity facilitates venous return, stroke volume is near maximal in the supine position. When comparing exercise responses in the upright and supine positions, heart rate and a-vO_2 difference are lower, but stroke volume and cardiac output are generally higher while supine (20,60). Thus, there is greater total blood flow and less oxygen extraction from the blood during supine versus upright exercise. However, the upright position may benefit tissue perfusion through an increase in driving force.

Static Versus Dynamic Exercise

Dynamic or **isotonic** exercise is defined as that in which movement through some range of motion occurs against gravity or the resistance of water. Most recreational exercises, such as walking, running, cycling, or swimming, generally fall into the isotonic category. In static or **isometric** exercise there is sustained muscle tension but no skeletal muscle movement, and muscle length remains constant, such as sustained hand grip or carrying a bag of groceries. Isometric exercise is much more stressful on the heart. Blood flow is mechanically impeded during sustained isometric muscle contraction, and the increase in cardiac output required for the exercise is accomplished with much greater increases in systolic and diastolic blood pressures than occur with a comparable level of isotonic exercise (61,62). Although left ventricular contractility increases, increases in stroke volume may be minimal. There is a moderate but widespread increase in vasoconstriction, caused by increased sympathetic nervous stimulation, although total systemic vascular resistance does not increase greatly (61). The increase in cardiac output is greater than the increase in oxygen uptake. The increased blood pressure increases afterload and myocardial pressure work, which results in a higher myocardial oxygen demand.

Strength training exercises require a greater degree of isometric than isotonic muscle contraction. The blood pressure response to isometric exercise is related to the comparatively smaller amount of muscle mass involved. Abdominal and thoracic pressures may increase considerably during lifting activities, particularly if an individual is not trained to lift and breathe properly. Although weight lifting under controlled conditions is now an accepted component of cardiac rehabilitation programs (63), these factors underscore the importance of proper supervision when including resistance exercises for patients with heart disease.

Prolonged Exercise

Clinically, the concern for patients with cardiovascular disease is most often the response to exercise testing, i.e., the measurement of cardiovascular function and exercise capacity, which is determined using an acute bout of exercise. The response to prolonged submaximal exercise differs considerably. Performance is related as much to substrate use, temperature regulation, and environmental factors as to cardiovascular function. Many studies have described progressive increases in heart rate and concomitant decreases in stroke volume during bouts of exercise that last longer than 30 min at intensities greater than 50% $\dot{V}O_2$max. This phenomenon has been called **cardiovascular drift** (64,65), in which the increase in heart rate counteracts the reduction in stroke volume to maintain cardiac output. It has been suggested that the progressive reduction in stroke volume during prolonged exercise is due to an increased core temperature resulting in a relative vasoconstriction in active skeletal muscle and displacement of blood volume to the cutaneous blood vessels (64,65). Decreases in central blood volume, pulmonary artery pressure, and filling pressure all appear to be part of the cardiovascular drift. Evidence exists that myocardial fatigue occurs with prolonged exercise, including changes in cardiac volumes, contractile function, and substrate use (65-68). However, not all studies agree on this issue (65). Thus, no convincing evidence exists that myocardial fatigue explains cardiovascular drift or that prolonged exercise causes any serious myocardial damage.

A relative increase in the use of fatty acids as a metabolic substrate occurs during prolonged exercise (69). The major factor limiting prolonged exercise appears to be the availability of muscle **glycogen** (69,70). One advantage conferred with exercise training is a greater reliance on fat as a substrate. The elevation in mitochondrial enzymes after training includes increases in enzymes for **beta-oxidation** of fats (71,72). This serves to spare muscle glycogen and improve endurance performance.

Factors Influencing Maximal Exercise Capacity

Factors that determine maximal exercise capacity and endurance performance have long attracted the attention of exercise scientists, and a great deal of effort continues in this area today. Clearly, the most influential factors are age, gender, and genetic endowment. While these factors are rather intuitive, the question more often concerns what limits subjects who are relatively homogeneous. For example, most athletes training in the same event are young, healthy, and genetically endowed, achieve high maximal cardiac output and oxygen uptake values, and have excellent cardiovascular health. Thus, predicting performance in these subjects presents a challenge. A similar problem exists among patients with cardiovascular disease. Limitations to exercise in patients with heart disease continue to intrigue cardiologists, since identifying limitations to exercise is a key factor in improving therapy. Following are reviews of the major factors that influence exercise capacity.

Cardiopulmonary Disease

Determining exercise capacity among patients with heart disease is more complicated than that in normal subjects. Determinants of exercise "impairment" rather than exercise performance are more often the focus of clinical studies. As in normals, $\dot{V}O_2$max is directly related to maximal cardiac output, and it is often assumed that exercise impairment directly reflects the degree of left ventricular dysfunction. This would appear to be supported by the general belief that the most important factor limiting $\dot{V}O_2$max in normals is the heart's ability to deliver oxygen (64,73).

However, the inability of central and peripheral factors to account for differences in exercise capacity in patients with heart disease has been perplexing. Patients often achieve levels of exercise discordant with their degree of cardiac disease that cannot be explained by disease in other organ systems. For example, a discrepancy between indices of left ventricular function and exercise capacity has been repeatedly observed, with correlation coefficients ranging from -0.10 to 0.24 between the two (17-19, 74-80) (see Figure 1.5 on p. 15). Although maximal heart rate, maximal cardiac output, and their change from rest to maximal exercise appear to account for the greatest variance in exercise capacity, they generally leave 50% or more of the variance in $\dot{V}O_2$max unexplained (17,77,78). The exercise response of patients with chronic heart failure is also affected by abnormalities in the pulmonary, neurohumoral, and skeletal muscle systems, in addition to their impaired cardiac function (18,74,75). Because specific mechanisms responsible for limiting exercise are often difficult to identify, therapy cannot be targeted to specific areas and clinical management of patients can be challenging. Recent studies among patients with chronically reduced ventricular function have demonstrated that programs of exercise training can improve a number of these abnormalities associated with exercise (81,82).

Patients with pulmonary disease similarly exhibit reduced exercise capacity, although the mechanisms differ. Abnormalities in the exchange of oxygen and carbon dioxide in the lungs can be caused by such things as reduced surface area for exchange, poor lung compliance, chronic obstruction to air flow, abnormal pulmonary mechanics, and abnormal pulmonary muscle function. In patients with severe lung disease, oxygen **desaturation** can occur during exercise. Some combination of these abnormalities leads to metabolic **acidosis** and breathlessness at low levels of exercise. Specific gas exchange responses of patients with cardiovascular and pulmonary disease are outlined in more detail in chapter 5.

Age

Among the most important factors influencing one's exercise capacity is age. Maximal oxygen uptake and age are inversely related: cross-sectional and longitudinal studies have shown that $\dot{V}O_2$max declines roughly 1% per year, although this varies considerably (83). Several studies have shown, however, that a decline in maximal oxygen uptake is not an obligatory consequence of aging; one's habitual physical activity level is a more important determinant of $\dot{V}O_2$max than age per se (84,85).

Gender

Females typically have $\dot{V}O_2$max values that are 15% to 30% below those of men, even among athletes or when matched by activity status (86-89). These differences have been explained by differences in body composition (greater ratio of fat weight to lean weight in women), smaller muscle mass, smaller cardiac output, smaller respiratory capacity, and lower hemoglobin levels. These factors probably combine to one extent or another to explain the differences in aerobic capacity between men and women.

Genetics

The role of natural endowment in cardiovascular function and exercise performance has long interested physiologists. Clearly, an exceptionally high aerobic capacity or the ability to compete at an elite level must reflect more than training. Indeed, among studies of paired identical and paired fraternal twins, heredity alone was reported to explain 93% of the observed differences in aerobic capacity (90,91). More recent studies have shown more modest but nevertheless major contributions of genetic factors to exercise performance (92,93). Ratios of muscle fiber types have been shown to be similar among identical twins, while fiber composition varies widely among fraternal twins or brothers (94). Both $\dot{V}O_2$max and the adaptations of most skeletal muscle enzymes to training appear to be largely genotype dependent (95-97).

Physical Training

Regular exercise increases work capacity. Hundreds of studies have been performed that document higher $\dot{V}O_2$max values among active versus sedentary individuals cross sectionally or when comparing groups after a period of training. The magnitude of the improvement in $\dot{V}O_2$max with training varies widely, generally ranging from 5% to 25%, but increases as large as 50% have been reported. The degree of change in $\dot{V}O_2$max is primarily dependent on initial state of fitness, but it is also affected by age and the type, frequency, and intensity of training. Although there are both peripheral (skeletal muscle) and central (cardiac) adaptations to training, the major adaptation that underlies an increase in $\dot{V}O_2$max is probably an increase in oxygen delivery via an enhanced end-diastolic volume and thus stroke volume and cardiac output (38,64). $\dot{V}O_2$max may range as low as 20 to 25 ml/kg/min in middle-aged sedentary individuals, although it is not uncommon to see patients with chronic heart failure achieve values less than 10 ml/kg/min (18,74). Values as high as 80 to 90 ml/kg/min have been observed among elite endurance athletes (98).

While $\dot{V}O_2$max is the best single measure of the limits of the cardiopulmonary system, it is clearly not the only determinant of endurance performance. In fact, $\dot{V}O_2$max varies widely for similar performances at the elite level. The physiological and biochemical factors that determine endurance performance have yet to be established. Factors other than $\dot{V}O_2$max, including the metabolic enzyme content of the skeletal muscles, running economy, the level of oxygen uptake before lactate accumulates in the blood, and psychological factors all contribute considerably to one's endurance performance.

Environment

Exercise responses have been extensively studied under conditions of heat, cold, and altitude and under different gravitational conditions. Under normal environmental conditions, body temperature, pH, and most metabolic processes are maintained within a narrow range, even with heavy exercise. In extreme environmental conditions, however, even mild exercise can disrupt the body's regulatory mechanisms. For example, up to 20% of distance runners suffer some form of heat illness as a result of prolonged exercise in hot, humid conditions (99,100). Environmental considerations can have an important impact not only on those concerned with athletic performance but also on cardiac rehabilitation. The following sections briefly review the effects of environmental conditions on the response to exercise.

Heat. During exercise in the heat, the distribution of cardiac output is faced with competing drives to provide the muscles with oxygen needed to sustain energy metabolism and to dissipate heat generated by metabolism from the muscle to the periphery (44,64,101). Thus, cutaneous and muscle blood flow is maintained at the expense of other tissues. However, mean arterial pressure and muscle blood flow appear to take precedence over temperature regulation (102). When dehydration accompanies prolonged exercise, less blood is directed to the skin for heat dissipation (103), perhaps reflecting an attempt to maintain cardiac output despite a reduced plasma volume as a result of sweating. Stroke volume is reduced (104,105), and compensatory increases have been observed in heart rate at any given submaximal level of exercise. In extreme cases, reductions in plasma volume can lead to circulatory failure, and core temperature may reach lethal levels. With training in the heat, acclimatization occurs, and the body is better able to sustain prolonged exercise in hot conditions. These adaptations include increases in blood volume, better core temperature regulation through earlier and more profuse sweating, and better skin vasodilatory capacity (101,106,107).

Cold. Because heat conduction is many times greater in water, cold water has been the major medium by which studies have evaluated exercise under hypothermic conditions. In contrast to responses to the heat, blood is shunted from the skin to the body core, and involuntary shivering may occur in an effort to increase metabolism. Oxygen uptake is higher and body temperature is lower in cold water compared with a matched intensity of exercise in warm water. The greater oxygen cost is a result of the added energy cost of shivering to counteract heat loss. The increase in metabolic rate due to cold can reduce work performance. This has particularly important implications for activity recommendations among patients with coronary artery disease; fluid shifts and increased metabolism caused by a cold environment can increase myocardial oxygen demand and lead to an increase in symptoms. Several studies have compared exercise testing responses in cold compared with normal laboratory environments and reported earlier and more pronounced angina and other signs of ischemia in the cold (108-110).

Altitude. Altitude causes a reduction in barometric pressure, resulting in a decrease in the partial pressure of oxygen in the ambient air (PO_2). Modest altitudes (4,000-6,000 feet, resulting in a 100 mmHg or more reduction in barometric pressure) may have little effect on an individual at rest, but measurable adverse effects on exercise performance may occur at altitudes as low as 4,000 feet (111). During the 1980s the response to exercise at high altitudes was described in an eloquent series of studies lead by John West and associates (112) on the slopes of Mt. Everest and in a decompression chamber in Natick, Massachusetts. The physiological effects of altitude at submaximal exercise levels include increases in ventilation, cardiac output, and heart rate, whereas $\dot{V}O_2$ and stroke volume are similar. At maximal exercise, oxygen uptake and heart rate are reduced. **Hyperventilation** causes a drop in PCO_2, and this respiratory **alkalosis** facilitates oxygen binding to hemoglobin in the pulmonary capillaries. Right heart catheterization studies at altitude have demonstrated pulmonary hypertension secondary to an increased pulmonary vascular resistance, lower right atrial pressure, and lower **pulmonary capillary wedge pressure** (113,114). Acclimatization to altitude includes (115)

- **polycythemia**;
- an increase in the hematocrit;
- an increase in 2,3-diphosphoglycerate facilitating a rightward shift in the oxyhemoglobin dissociation curve; and
- increases in skeletal muscle capillary number, mitochondria, oxidative enzymes, and **myoglobin**.

Interestingly, these adaptations do not appear to confer any major advantages for performance at sea level (116-118).

SUMMARY

This chapter provided an overview of basic exercise physiology with the focus on cardiopulmonary adaptations to exercise. Exercise testing is a common and very practical test during which total body oxygen uptake can be measured directly and cardiac perfusion and function can be assessed indirectly. The physiologic adaptations that occur in response to exercise make it an important tool not only for the study of the limits of human performance in athletes but also for the study of cardiovascular and pulmonary disease. The exercise test in effect quantifies the limits of work under controlled conditions. "Work" is an important concept, but the many ways in which it is expressed have led to some confusion.

The common biological measure of work is total body oxygen uptake, expressed in liters per minute. The measurement of the body's physiologic work is most accurately performed directly with the use of gas exchange techniques. Estimating exercise capacity by treadmill or cycle ergometer time or workload achieved is common clinically, but it is less precise and less reproducible. The evaluation of exercise capacity is an important component of an exercise test clinically, as it provides data that have important functional, diagnostic, and prognostic implications. It also provides the foundation for developing an exercise prescription.

With maximal exercise, oxygen uptake can increase as much as 5 to 20 times its resting value. The degree to which oxygen uptake increases depends on the type of exercise performed, the presence of cardiovascular or pulmonary disease, age, gender, and fitness of the individual. Maximal oxygen uptake is defined as the product of maximal cardiac output and maximal arteriovenous oxygen difference. Thus, the cardiopulmonary limits are defined by a central component (cardiac output), which describes the capacity of the heart to function as a pump, and peripheral factors (arteriovenous oxygen difference), which describe the capacity of the lung to oxygenate the blood delivered to it and the capacity of the working muscle to extract this oxygen from the blood.

REFERENCES

1. Sullivan M, McKirnan MD. 1984. Errors in predicting functional capacity for postmyocardial infarction patients using a modified Bruce protocol. Am Heart J 107: 486-491.
2. Roberts JM, Sullivan M, Froelicher VF, Genter F, Myers J. 1984. Predicting oxygen uptake from treadmill testing in normal subjects and coronary artery disease patients. Am Heart J 108: 1454-1460.
3. Myers J, Buchanan N, Walsh D, Kraemer M, McAuley P, Hamilton-Wessler M, Froelicher VF. 1991. Comparison of the ramp versus standard exercise protocols. J Am Coll Cardiol 17: 1334-1342.

4. Petersen ES, Whipp BJ, Davis JA, Huntsman DJ, Brown HV, Wasserman K. 1983. Effects of *b*-adrenergic blockade on ventilation and gas exchange during exercise in humans. J Appl Physiol 54: 1306-1313.
5. Hughson RL, Russell CA, Marshall MR. 1984. Effect of metoprolol on cycle and treadmill maximal exercise performance. J Cardiac Rehabil 4: 27-30.
6. Haskell W, Savin W, Oldridge N, DeBusk R. 1982. Factors influencing estimated oxygen uptake during exercise testing soon after myocardial infarction. Am J Cardiol 50: 299-304.
7. Starling MR, Moody M, Crawford MH, Levi B, O'Rourke RA. 1984. Repeat treadmill exercise testing: Variability of results in patients with angina pectoris. Am Heart J 107: 298-303.
8. Elborn JS, Stanford CF, Nichols DP. 1990. Reproducibility of cardiopulmonary parameters during exercise in patients with chronic cardiac failure: The need for a preliminary test. Eur Heart J 11: 75-81.
9. Pinsky DJ, Ahern D, Wilson PB, Kukin ML, Packer M. 1989. How many exercise tests are needed to minimize the placebo effect of serial exercise testing in patients with chronic heart failure? Circulation 80 (suppl II): II-426.
10. Sullivan M, Genter F, Savvides M, Roberts M, Myers J, Froelicher VF. 1984. The reproducibility of hemodynamic, electrocardiographic, and gas exchange data during treadmill exercise in patients with stable angina pectoris. Chest 86: 375-382.
11. American College of Sports Medicine. 1995. Guidelines for Exercise Testing and Exercise Prescription, 5th ed. Philadelphia: Lea and Febiger.
12. Noakes TD. 1988. Implications of exercise testing for prediction of athletic performance: A contemporary perspective. Med Sci Sports Exerc 20: 319-330.
13. Myers J, Walsh D, Buchanan N, Froelicher VF. 1989. Can maximal cardiopulmonary capacity be recognized by a plateau in oxygen uptake? Chest 96: 1312-1316.
14. Myers J, Walsh D, Sullivan M, Froelicher VF. 1990. Effect of sampling on variability and plateau in oxygen uptake. J Appl Physiol 68 (1): 404-410.
15. Hammond HK, Froelicher VF. 1985. Normal and abnormal heart rate responses to exercise. Prog Cardiovasc Dis 27 (4): 271-296.
16. Froelicher VF, Myers J, Follansbee WP, Labovitz AJ. 1993. Exercise and the Heart, 3d ed. St. Louis: Mosby-Year Book.
17. McKirnan MD, Sullivan M, Jensen D, Froelicher VF. 1984. Treadmill performance and cardiac function in selected patients with coronary heart disease. J Am Coll Cardiol 3: 253-261.
18. Myers J, Froelicher VF. 1991. Hemodynamic determinants of exercise capacity in chronic heart failure. Ann Intern Med 115: 377-386.
19. Franciosa JA, Park M, Levine TB. 1981. Lack of correlation between exercise capacity and indexes of resting left ventricular performance in heart failure. Am J Cardiol 47: 33-39.

20. Poliner LR, Dehmer GJ, Lewis SE, Parkey RW, Blomqvist CG, Willerson JT. 1980. Left ventricular performance in normal subjects: A comparison of the responses to exercise in the upright and supine positions. Circulation 62: 528-534.

21. Manyeri DE, Kostuk WJ. 1983. Right and left ventricular function at rest and during bicycle exercise in the supine and sitting positions in normal subjects and patients with coronary artery disease. Assessment by radionuclide ventriculography. Am J Cardiol 51: 36-42.

22. Higginbotham MB, Morris KG, Williams RS, McHale PA, Coleman RE, Cobb FR. 1986. Regulation of stroke volume during submaximal and maximal upright exercise in normal man. Circ Res 58: 281-291.

23. Rerych SK, Scholz PM, Newman GE, Sabiston DC Jr, Jones RH. 1978. Cardiac function at rest and during exercise in normals and in patients with coronary heart disease. Evaluation by radionuclide angiography. Ann Surg 187: 449-464.

24. Iskandrian AS, Hakki AH. 1986. Determinants of the changes in left ventricular end-diastolic volume during upright exercise in patients with coronary artery disease. Am Heart J 112: 441-446.

25. Wyns W, Melin JA, Vanbutsele RJ, DeCoster PM, Steels M, Piret L, Detry JMR. 1982. Assessment of right and left ventricular volumes during upright exercise in normal men. Eur Heart J 3: 529-536.

26. Renlund DG, Lakatta EG, Fleg JL, Becher LC, Clulow JF, Weisfeldt ML, Gerstenblith G. 1987. Prolonged decrease in cardiac volumes after maximal upright bicycle exercise. J Appl Physiol 63: 1947-1955.

27. Plotnick GD, Becker L, Fisher ML, Gerstenblith G, Renlund DG, Fleg JL, Weisfeldt ML, Lakatta EG. 1986. Use of the Frank-Starling mechanism during submaximal versus maximal upright exercise. Am J Physiol 251: H1101-H1105.

28. Ginzton LE, Conant R, Brizendine M, Laks MM. 1989. Effect of long-term high intensity aerobic training on left ventricular volume during maximal upright exercise. J Am Coll Cardiol 14: 364-371.

29. Freeman MR, Berman DS, Staniloff H, ElKayam V, Maddahi J, Swan HJC, Forrester J. 1981. Comparison of upright and supine bicycle exercise in the detection and evaluation of extent of coronary artery disease by equilibrium radionuclide ventriculography. Am Heart J 102: 182-189.

30. Shen WF, Roubin GS, Choong CY-P, Hutton BF, Harris PJ, Fletcher PJ, Kelley DT. 1985. Left ventricular response to exercise in coronary artery disease: Relation to myocardial ischemia and effects of nifedipine. Eur Heart J 6: 1025-1031.

31. Kalisher AL, Johnson LL, Johnson YE, Stone J, Feder JL, Escala E, Cannon PJ. 1984. Effects of propranolol and timolol on left ventricular volumes during exercise in patients with coronary artery disease. J Am Coll Cardiol 3: 210-218.

32. Sullivan MJ, Higginbotham MB, Cobb FR. 1988. Exercise training in patients with severe left ventricular dysfunction. Hemodynamic and metabolic effects. Circulation 78: 506-515.

33. Hakki AH, Iskandrian AS. 1985. Determinants of exercise capacity in patients with coronary artery disease: Clinical implications. J Cardiac Rehabil 5: 341-348.
34. Crawford MH, Petru MA, Rabinowitz C. 1985. Effect of isotonic exercise training on left ventricular volume during upright exercise. Circulation 72: 1237-1243.
35. Myers J, Wallis J, Lehmann K, Graettinger W, Waibel W, Froelicher VF. 1991. Hemodynamic determinants of maximal ventilatory oxygen uptake in patients with coronary artery disease. Circulation 84: II-150.
36. Andersen P, Henriksson J. 1977. Capillary supply of the quadriceps femoris muscle of man: Adaptive response to exercise. J Physiol (London) 270: 677-691.
37. Saltin B, Gollnick PD. 1983. Skeletal muscle adaptability: Significance for metabolism and performance. In LD Peachy, RH Adrian, SR Geiger, eds. Handbook of Physiology, Section 10, Skeletal Muscle, pp. 555-631. Bethesda, MD: American Physiological Society.
38. Saltin B, Rowell LB. 1980. Functional adaptations to physical activity and inactivity. Fed Proc 39: 1506-1516.
39. Blomqvist CG. 1982. Similarity of the hemodynamic responses to static and dynamic exercise of small muscle groups. Circ Res 48 (suppl I): 87-91.
40. Lewis SF. 1983. Cardiovascular responses to exercise as functions of absolute and relative work load. J Appl Physiol 54: 1314-1319.
41. Hermanson L, Saltin B. 1969. Oxygen uptake during maximal treadmill and bicycle exercise. J Appl Physiol 26: 31-37.
42. Buchfuhrer MJ, Hansen JE, Robinson TE, Sue DY, Wasserman K, Whipp BJ. 1983. Optimizing the exercise protocol for cardiopulmonary assessment. J Appl Physiol 55: 1558-1564.
43. Toner MN. 1983. Cardiorespiratory responses to exercise distributed between the upper and lower body. J Appl Physiol 54: 1403-1408.
44. Rowell LB. 1974. Human cardiovascular adjustments to exercise and thermal stress. Physiol Rev 54: 75-159.
45. Balady GJ, Schick EC, Weiner DA, Ryan TJ. 1986. Comparison of determinants of myocardial oxygen consumption during arm and leg exercise in normal persons. Am J Cardiol 57: 1385-1387.
46. Vokac Z, Bell H, Bautz-Holter E. 1975. Oxygen uptake/heart rate relationship in leg and arm exercise, sitting and standing. J Appl Physiol 39 (1): 54-59.
47. Louhevaara V, Sovijarvi A, Ilmarinen J, Teraslinna P. 1990. Differences in cardiorespiratory responses during and after arm crank and cycle exercise. Acta Physiol Scand 138: 133-143.
48. Magel JR, Faulkner JA. 1967. Maximum oxygen uptake of college swimmers. J Appl Physiol 22: 929.
49. Magel JR, Foglia GF, McArdle WD, Gutin B. 1975. Specificity of swim training on maximum oxygen uptake. J Appl Physiol 38: 151.

50. Hagberg JM, Giese MD, Schneider RB. 1978. Comparison of three procedures for measuring $\dot{V}O_2$max in competitive cyclists. Eur J Appl Physiol 39: 47.
51. Stromme SB, Ingjer F, Meem HD. 1977. Assessment of maximal aerobic power in specially trained athletes. J Appl Physiol 42: 833-837.
52. Myers J, Froelicher VF. 1990. Optimizing the exercise test for pharmacological investigations. Circulation 82: 1839-1846.
53. Webster MWI, Sharpe DN. 1989. Exercise testing in angina pectoris: The importance of protocol design in clinical trials. Am Heart J 117: 505-508.
54. Panza JA, Quyyumi AA, Diodati JG, Callaham TS, Epstein SE. 1991. Prediction of the frequency and duration of ambulatory myocardial ischemia in patients with stable coronary artery disease by determination of the ischemic threshold from exercise testing: Importance of the exercise protocol. J Am Coll Cardiol 17: 657-663.
55. Garber CE, Carleton RA, Camaione DN, Heller GV. 1991. The threshold for myocardial ischemia varies in patients with coronary artery disease depending on the exercise protocol. J Am Coll Cardiol 17: 1256-1262.
56. Myers J, Buchanan N, Smith D, Neutel J, Bowes E, Walsh D, Froelicher VF. 1991. Individualized ramp treadmill: Observations on a new protocol. Chest 101: 2305-2415.
57. Haskell W, Savin W, Oldridge N, DeBusk R. 1982. Factors influencing estimated oxygen uptake during exercise testing soon after myocardial infarction. Am J Cardiol 50: 299-304.
58. Tamesis B, Stelken A, Byers S, Shaw L, Younis L, Miller D, Chaitman BR. 1993. Comparison of the asymptomatic cardiac ischemia pilot and modified asymptomatic cardiac ischemia pilot versus Bruce and Cornell Exercise Protocols. Am J Cardiol 72: 715-720.
59. Redwood DR, Rosing DR, Goldstein RE, Beiser GD, Epstein SE. 1971. Importance of the design of an exercise protocol in the evaluation of patients with angina pectoris. Circulation 43: 618-628.
60. Bevegard S, Holmgren A, Jonsson B. 1963. Circulatory studies in well-trained athletes at rest and during heavy exercise, with special reference to stroke volume and the influence of body position. Acta Physiol Scand 57 (1-2): 26-50.
61. Lind AR. 1983. Cardiovascular adjustments to isometric contractions: Static effort. In JR Shepherd, FM Abbound, eds. Handbook of Physiology, Section 2, Volume III, Peripheral Circulation, Part 2, pp. 947-966. Bethesda, MD: American Physiological Society.
62. Nutter DO, Schland RC, Hurst JW. 1972. Isometric exercise and the cardiovascular system. Mod Concepts Cardiovasc Dis 41 (3): 11-15.
63. American Association of Cardiovascular and Pulmonary Rehabilitation. 1995. Guidelines for Cardiac Rehabilitation Programs, 2d ed. Champaign, IL: Human Kinetics.
64. Rowell LB. 1986. Human Circulation: Regulation During Physical Stress, 257-286, 308-322, 356-374. New York: Oxford Press.

65. Raven PB, Stevens GHJ. 1988. Cardiovascular function and prolonged exercise. In DR Lamb, R Murray, eds. Prolonged Exercise, 43-74. Indianapolis: Benchmark Press.
66. Saltin B, Stenberg J. 1964. Circulatory responses to prolonged severe exercise. J Appl Physiol 19 (5): 833-838.
67. Upton MT, Rerych SK, Roeback JR Jr, Newman GE, Douglas JM Jr, Wallace AG, Jones RH. 1980. Effect of brief and prolonged exercise on left ventricular function. Am J Cardiol 45: 1154-1160.
68. Niemela KO, Palatsi IJ, Ikaheimo MJ, Takkunen JT, Vuori JJ. 1984. Evidence of impaired left ventricular performance after an interrupted competitive 24-hour run. Circulation 70 (3): 350-356.
69. Gollnick PD. 1988. Energy metabolism and prolonged exercise. In DR Lamb, R Murray, eds. Prolonged Exercise, 1-42. Indianapolis: Benchmark Press.
70. Heigenhauser GJF, Sutton JR, Jones NL. 1983. Effect of glycogen depletion on the ventilatory response to exercise. J Appl Physiol 54: 470-474.
71. Gollnick PD, Pernow B, Essen B, Jansson E, Saltin B. 1981. Availability of glycogen and plasma FFA for substrate utilization in leg muscle of man during exercise. Clin Physiol 1: 27-42.
72. Gollnick PD, Riedy M, Quintinskie JJ, Bertocci LA. 1985. Differences in metabolic potential of skeletal muscle fibers and their significance for metabolic control. J Exp Biol 115: 191-199.
73. diPrampero PE. 1985. Metabolic and circulatory limitations to $\dot{V}O_2$max at the whole animal level. J Exp Biol 115: 319-331.
74. Szlachcic J, Massie BM, Kramer BL, Topic N, Tubau J. 1985. Correlates and prognostic implication of exercise capacity in chronic congestive heart failure. Am J Cardiol 55: 1037-1042.
75. Massie BM. 1988. Exercise tolerance in congestive heart failure. Role of cardiac function, peripheral blood flow, and muscle metabolism and effect of treatment. Am J Med 84: 75-82.
76. Baker JB, Wilen MM, Body CM, Dinh H, Franciosa JA. 1984. Relation of right ventricular ejection fraction to exercise capacity in chronic left ventricular failure. Am J Cardiol 54: 596-599.
77. Meller SE, Ashton JJ, Moeschberger ML, Unverferth DV, Leier CV. 1987. An analysis of the determinants of exercise performance in congestive heart failure. Am Heart J 113: 1207-1217.
78. Higginbotham MB, Morris KG, Conn EH, Coleman RE, Cobb FR. 1983. Determinants of variable exercise performance among patients with severe left ventricular dysfunction. Am J Cardiol 51: 52-60.
79. Franciosa JA, Leddy CL, Wilen M, Schwartz DE. 1984. Relation between hemodynamic and ventilatory responses in determining exercise capacity in severe congestive heart failure. Am J Cardiol 53: 127-134.
80. Myers J, Salleh A, Buchanan N, Smith D, Neutel J, Bowes E, Froelicher VF. 1992. Ventilatory mechanisms of exercise intolerance in chronic heart failure. Am Heart J 124: 710-719.

81. Coats AJS, Adamopolous S, Radaeli A, McCance A, Meyer TE, Bernardi L, Solda PL, Davey P, Ormerod O, Forfar C, Conway J, Sleight P. 1992. Controlled trial of physical training in chronic heart failure. Exercise performance, hemodynamics, ventilation, and autonomic function. Circulation 85: 2119-2131.

82. Sullivan MJ, Higginbotham MB, Cobb FR. 1988. Exercise training in patients with severe left ventricular function. Hemodynamic and metabolic effects. Circulation 78: 506-515.

83. Åstrand PO, Rodahl K. 1986. Textbook of Work Physiology, 3d ed. New York: McGraw-Hill.

84. Meredith CN, Zackin MJ, Frontera WR, Evans WJ. 1987. Body composition and aerobic capacity in young and middle-aged endurance-trained men Med Sci Sports Exerc 19: 557-563.

85. Upton SJ, Hagan RD, Lease B, Rosentswieg J, Gettman LR, Duncan JJ. 1984. Comparative physiological profiles among young and middle-aged female distance runners. Med Sci Sports Exerc 16: 67-71.

86. Vogel JA, Patton JF, Mello RP, Daniels WL. 1986. An analysis of aerobic capacity in a large United States population. J Appl Physiol 60: 494.

87. Hansen JE, Sue DY, Wasserman K. 1984. Predicted values for clinical exercise testing. Am Rev Respir Dis 129 (suppl): 549-555.

88. Hermansen LH, Anderson L. 1965. Aerobic work capacity in young Norwegian men and women. J Appl Physiol 20: 425.

89. Vergh V. 1987. The influence of body mass in cross-country skiing. Med Sci Sports Exerc 19: 324-344.

90. Klissouras V. 1971. Heritability of adaptive variation. J Appl Physiol 31: 338.

91. Klissouras V, Pirnay F, Petit JM. 1973. Adaptation to maximal effort: Genetics and age. J Appl Physiol 35: 288-293, 1973.

92. Bouchard C, Lortie J. 1984. Heredity and human performance. Sports Med 1: 38.

93. Bouchard C, Lesage R, Lortie G, Simoneau JA. 1986. Aerobic performance in brothers, dizygotic and monozygotic twins. Med Sci Sports Exerc 18: 639-646.

94. Lortie G. 1986. Muscle fiber type composition and enzyme activities in brothers and monozygotic twins. In RM Malina, C Bouchard, eds. Proceedings of the 1984 Olympic Scientific Congress, Volume 4. Sport and Human Genetics. Champaign, IL: Human Kinetics.

95. Bouchard C. 1986. Genetic effects in human skeletal muscle fiber type distribution and enzyme activities. Can J Physiol Pharmacol 64: 125.

96. Hammel P, Simoneau JA, Lortie G, Boulay MR, Bouchard C. 1986. Heredity and muscle adaptation to endurance training. Med Sci Sports Exerc 18: 690-696.

97. Prud'homme D, Bouchard C, LeBlanc C, Landry F, Fontaine E. 1984. Sensitivity of maximal aerobic power to training is genotype-dependent. Med Sci Sports Exerc 16: 489-493.

98. Pollock ML. 1977. Submaximal and maximal working capacity of elite distance runners. Part I: Cardiorespiratory aspects. Ann NY Acad Sci 301: 310-321.
99. Hanson PG. 1979. Heat injury in runners. Phys Sportsmedicine 7: 91-96.
100. Hughson RL, Green JH, Houston ME, Thomson JA, MacLean DR, Sutton JR. 1980. Heat injuries in Canadian mass participation runs. Can Med Assoc J 122: 1141-1144.
101. Brengelmann GL. 1983. Circulatory adjustments to exercise and heat stress. Annu Rev Physiol 45: 191-212.
102. Nadel ER, Cafarelli E, Roberts MF, Wenger CB. 1979. Circulatory regulation during exercise in different ambient temperatures. J Appl Physiol 46: 430-437.
103. Fortney SM, Wenger CB, Bove JR, Nadel ER. 1984. Effect of hyperosmolarity on control of blood flow and sweating. J Appl Physiol 57: 1668-1695.
104. Robinson S. 1965. Acclimatization of older men to work in the heat. J Appl Physiol 20: 583-588.
105. Williams CG. 1962. Circulatory and metabolic reactions to work in heat. J Appl Physiol 17: 625-630.
106. Gisolfi CV, Wenger CB. 1984. Temperature regulation during exercise: Old concepts, new ideas. Exerc Sport Sci Rev 12: 339-372.
107. Harrison MH. 1985. Effects of thermal stress and exercise in blood volume in humans. Physiol Rev 65 (1): 149-209.
108. Juneau M, Johnstone M, Dempsey E, Waters DD. 1989. Exercise-induced myocardial ischemia in a cold environment: Effect of antianginal medications. Circulation 79: 1015-1020.
109. Lassvik CT, Areskog N. 1979. Angina in cold environment: Reactions to exercise. Br Heart J 42: 396-401.
110. Shea MJ, Deanfield JE, deLandsheere CM, Wilson RA, Kensett M, Selwyn AP. 1987. Asymptomatic ischemia following cold provocation. Am Heart J 114: 469-476.
111. Squires RW, Buskirk ER. 1982. Aerobic capacity during acute exposure to simulated altitude, 914 to 2,286 meters. Med Sci Sports Exerc 14: 36-41.
112. West JB, Boyer JJ, Graber DJ, Hackett PH, Maret KH, Milledge JS, Peters RM, Pizzo CJ, Samaja M, Sarnquist FH, Schoene RB, Winslow RM. 1983. Maximal exercise at extreme altitudes on Mount Everest. J Appl Physiol 55: 678-687.
113. Groves BM, Reeves JT, Sutton JR, Wagner PD. 1987. Operation Everest II: Elevated high-altitude pulmonary resistance unresponsive to oxygen. J Appl Physiol 63: 521-530.
114. Reeves JT, Groves BM, Sutton JR, Wagner PD. 1987. Operation Everest II: Preservation of cardiac function at extreme altitude. J Appl Physiol 63: 531-539.
115. Young AJ, Young PM. 1988. Human acclimatization to high terrestrial altitude. In KB Pandolf, ed. Human Performance Physiology and Environmental Medicine at Terrestrial Extremes. Indianapolis: Benchmark Press.

116. Balke B. 1966. Effects of altitude acclimatization on work capacity. Fed Proc 15: 7-17.
117. Buskirk ER, Kollias J, Akers RF, Prokop EK, Reategui EP. 1967. Maximal performance at altitude and on return from altitude in conditioned runners. J Appl Physiol 23: 259-266.
118. Mizuno M, Juel C, Bro-Rasmussen T, Mygind E. 1990. Limb skeletal muscle adaptation in athletes after training at altitude. J Appl Physiol 68: 496-502.

CHAPTER
2

PRINCIPLES OF
EXERCISE TESTING

*T*he many approaches to exercise testing have been a drawback to its proper application: agreement on how the test should be performed is lacking. Not surprisingly, gas exchange techniques introduce several additional factors that can potentially complicate methodology. Specific principles of gas exchange techniques are discussed in forthcoming chapters. The inconsistencies over methodology have been improved by excellent guidelines that have recently been updated by organizations such as the American Heart Association (AHA), the American Association of Cardiovascular and Pulmonary Rehabilitation (AACVPR), and the American College of Sports Medicine (ACSM) (1-3). These guidelines have evolved from a multitude of research studies over the last 20 years and have led to greater uniformity in methods. Nevertheless, in many laboratories, methodology remains based on tradition, convenience, equipment, or personnel available.

Recent technology, while adding convenience, has raised new questions about methodology. Increased automation has permitted greater use of ventilatory gas exchange techniques, leading to improved precision in the measurement of work. However, these advances in gas exchange systems require additional knowledge by the user to assure that the data acquired are valid. In addition, nearly all commercially available ECG systems today include computers. While this has certainly made things easier, questions remain as to how computer-averaged ECGs or the newer computer/ exercise scores influence test performance (3). The present chapter will address these issues and other basic principles and methods for standard exercise testing. The major methodologic concerns include appropriate indications, personnel and other safety issues, testing protocols, measurement and interpretation of hemodynamic responses, and interpretation of the exercise electrocardiogram.

METHODOLOGIC CONSIDERATIONS

The key methodologic considerations include exercise testing indications, personnel, the exercise protocol and mode, contraindications, the electrocardiogram, test interpretation, and patient safety issues.

Indications for Exercise Testing

The exercise test can have a wide range of clinical applications, and the indications for its use have increased over the years. Nevertheless, while the diagnostic and prognostic information from the test is valuable in some patients, it is not very useful in some individuals, and the test is contraindicated in others. A recent joint task force on exercise testing has divided indications for exercise testing into three classes based on the likely information yield (4). The American College of Sports Medicine has outlined indications for exercise testing based on age, gender, and presenting symptoms (2). General indications for testing are presented in Table 2.1.

Exercise Testing Personnel

In 1990, a joint statement was issued by the American College of Physicians (ACP), the American College of Cardiology (ACC), and the American Heart Association (AHA) regarding physician competence in exercise testing (4). This was the first position statement of its type. The necessary cognitive skills needed to perform exercise testing, which were outlined in this statement, included knowledge of indications and contraindications to testing, basic exercise physiology, principles of interpretation, and emergency procedures. The committee suggested that at least 50 procedures were required during training. Likewise, technicians should have familiarity with these basic skills. The ACSM has developed certification programs for competency in exercise testing and training (2).

Table 2.1   Indications for Exercise Testing

- Evaluating chest pain
- Screening for ischemic heart disease in at-risk asymptomatic males
- Evaluating dysrhythmias
- Determining functional capacity
- Generating an exercise prescription
- Establishing the severity/prognosis of ischemic heart disease to stratify those who need additional intervention, that is, angioplasty versus coronary artery bypass graft (CABG)
- Evaluating antianginal or antihypertensive therapy
- Evaluating antiarrhythmic therapy
- Evaluating the patient after myocardial infarction for risk stratification

---

ACSM certification is strongly recommended for technicians, nurses, or physiologists who oversee exercise testing and training. Because surveys have shown that complications during exercise testing are extremely rare, particularly in recent years (5,6), the question has been raised as to whether physician supervision is required for all exercise testing (7). Most authorities continue to feel that physician presence is required when testing individuals with cardiovascular or pulmonary disease or those who are at high risk for developing disease. The ACSM has also outlined general guidelines where physician supervision is recommended (2). Needless to say, proper administration and application of gas exchange techniques require an additional degree of expertise by both the physician and technician.

Exercise Protocols

Protocols can differ considerably in terms of the rate at which work is incremented and the duration of time between stages. This has led to some confusion regarding how physicians compare tests between patients and serial tests in the same patient. Some common protocols, their stages, and the predicted oxygen cost of each stage are illustrated in Figure 2.1. When treadmill testing and cycle ergometer testing were first introduced into clinical practice, practitioners adopted protocols used by major researchers such as Balke (8), Åstrand (9), Bruce (10), and Ellestad (11) and their respective co-workers. In 1980, Stuart and Ellestad (12) surveyed 1,375 exercise laboratories in North America and reported that of those performing treadmill testing, 65.5% used the Bruce protocol for routine clinical testing. Since then, an appreciation for more gradual, individualized approaches has occurred (such as modifications of the Balke or ramp-type protocols) (3,13-20). Arguments in favor of more gradual approaches come from several directions. Large and unequal work increments have been shown to result in less accurate estimates

FUNCTIONAL CLASS	CLINICAL STATUS	O₂ COST ml/kg/min	METS	BICYCLE ERGOMETER 1 WATT = 6.1 Kpm/min (FOR 70 KG BODY WEIGHT) Kpm/min	BRUCE 3 MIN STAGES MPH / %GR	BALKE-WARE % GRADE AT 3.3 MPH, 1 MIN STAGES	USAFSAM MPH / %GR	"SLOW" USAFSAM MPH / %GR	McHENRY MPH / %GR	STANFORD % GRADE AT 3 MPH	STANFORD % GRADE AT 2 MPH	ACIP MPH / %GR	CHF MPH / %GR	METS
NORMAL AND I	HEALTHY, DEPENDENT ON AGE, ACTIVITY	56.0	16		5.5 / 20	26								16
		52.5	15		5.0 / 18	25	3.3 / 25							15
		49.0	14			24, 23								14
		45.5	13	1500	4.2 / 16	22, 21	3.3 / 20							13
		42.0	12	1350		20, 19								12
	SEDENTARY HEALTHY	38.5	11	1200		18, 17	3.3 / 15		3.3 / 21	22.5		3.4 / 24.0		11
		35.0	10	1050	3.4 / 14	16, 15			3.3 / 18	20.0		3.1 / 24.0	3.4 / 14.0	10
		31.5	9	900		14, 13	3.3 / 10	2 / 25	3.3 / 15	17.5		3.0 / 21.0	3.0 / 15.0	9
		28.0	8			12, 11		2 / 20	3.3 / 12	15.0		3.0 / 17.5	3.0 / 12.5	8
		24.5	7	750	2.5 / 12	10, 9	3.3 / 5	2 / 15	3.3 / 9	12.5	17.5	3.0 / 14.0	3.0 / 10.0	7
		21.0	6	600		8, 7		2 / 10	3.3 / 6	10.0	14.0	3.0 / 10.5	3.0 / 7.5	6
II		17.5	5	450	1.7 / 10	6, 5	3.3 / 0	2 / 5		7.5	10.5	3.0 / 7.0	2.0 / 10.5	5
III	LIMITED	14.0	4	300	1.7 / 5	4, 3				5.0	7.0	3.0 / 3.0	2.0 / 7.0	4
		10.5	3	150	1.7 / 0	2, 1	2.0 / 0	2 / 0	2.0 / 3	2.5	3.5	2.5 / 2.0	2.0 / 3.5	3
IV	SYMPTOMATIC	7.0	2							0		2.0 / 0.0	1.5 / 0.0	2
		3.5	1										1.0 / 0.0	1

USAFSAM = United States Air Force School of Aerospace Medicine
ACIP = Asymptomatic Cardiac Ischemia Pilot
CHF = Congestive Heart Failure (Modified Naughton)
Kpm/min = Kilopond meters/minute
%GR = percent grade
MPH = miles per hour

Figure 2.1 The oxygen cost per stage of some commonly used protocols.

of exercise capacity, particularly for patients with cardiac disease. Recent investigations have demonstrated that work rate increments that are too large or rapid result in

- a tendency to overestimate exercise capacity (14,15,21),
- less reliability for studying the effects of therapy (16,18,19), and
- lowered sensitivity for detecting coronary disease (22).

Individualizing the protocol, considering the subject and purpose of the test, rather than employing the same protocol for every subject, appears to offer several advantages for cardiopulmonary assessment.

Protocols suitable for clinical testing should include a low-intensity warm-up phase followed by progressive, continuous exercise in which the demand is elevated to a patient's maximal level within a total duration of 8 to 12 min. Tests of this duration are recommended because they have been shown to optimize the information yield from the test: the highest values for maximal oxygen uptake are achieved, the relationship between measured and predicted oxygen uptake is closest, and it is most suitable for evaluating the effects of therapy (13,15,16,18,19). In the absence of gas exchange techniques, it is important to report exercise capacity in predicted METs rather than treadmill time, so that exercise capacity can be compared uniformly between protocols. METs can be estimated from any protocol using standardized equations that have been put into tabular form (2,3) (Figure 2.1). For patients with cardiovascular disease, modifications of the Balke-Ware protocol are often recommended because of its constant treadmill speed between 2 and 3.3 mph, equal increments in grade (2.5% or 5%), and equal (one or two) increases in METs.

When testing athletes, the protocol should also be individualized and an 8- to 12-min duration is optimal. The increments in work should be adapted in accordance with the subject's level of fitness. Training specificity should be considered; that is, the athlete will perform better when tested using an exercise mode for which he or she is trained. For runners, we have used an individualized protocol that begins with a short period of walking, increasing gradually to the subject's typical running pace by the 3rd or 4th min, followed by 2.5% or 5% increases in grade every 2 min until exhaustion. This virtually ensures a test duration of roughly 8 to 12 min and usually avoids the steeper treadmill grades (> 15%) in which back discomfort and awkwardness frequently cause a tendency to hold onto the handrails. A running protocol negates accurate ECG and blood pressure recordings, so the subjects' health must be ascertained beforehand. Other reasonable choices for fit individuals are the Bruce (10) and Ellestad (11) protocols. Many of the newer cycle ergometers have ramp controllers, in which a watts/minute rate can be specified. A suitable incremental protocol for healthy individuals who cycle routinely is roughly 50 watts in 2- or 3-min stages, similar to that described by Åstrand (9).

An approach to exercise testing that has drawn interest in recent years is the ramp protocol, in which work increases continuously. In 1981, Whipp and co-workers (59) first described cardiopulmonary responses to a ramp test on a cycle ergometer, and several gas exchange manufacturers now include ramp software.

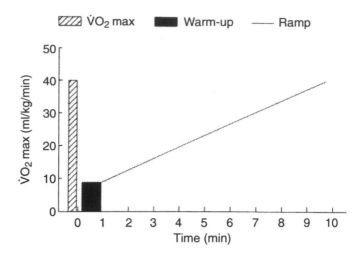

Figure 2.2   The ramp treadmill test. Following a 1-min warm-up at 2.0 mph/0% grade, the rate of change in speed and grade is individualized to yield the work rate (X axis) corresponding to maximal oxygen uptake (Y axis, obtained from the baseline test) in 10 min. Reprinted from Myers et al. 1992.

Recently, treadmills have also been adapted to conduct ramp tests (15,17) (Figure 2.2). The recent call for "optimizing" exercise testing (13-20) would appear to be facilitated by the ramp approach, since large work increments are avoided. Moreover, because it allows for increases in work to be individualized, a given test duration can be targeted.

By comparing gas exchange responses with commonly used protocols, we have observed that ramp tests with the work rate individualized yield the most accurate estimate of exercise capacity (15). The relationships between oxygen uptake and work rate (predicted oxygen uptake), defined as a slope for each of six protocols, were presented in chapter 1 (Table 1.3). These relationships, which reflect the degree of change in oxygen uptake for a given increase in work (a slope of unity would suggest that the cardiopulmonary system is adapting in direct accordance with the demands of the work), were highest for the ramp tests and lowest for the protocols containing the greatest increments in work. Further, the variance about the slope (SEE in oxygen uptake, ml/kg/min) was largest for the tests with the largest increments between stages (Bruce treadmill and 50 watts/stage bicycle) and smallest for the ramp tests. These observations suggest that oxygen uptake is overestimated from tests that contain large increments in work and the variability in estimating oxygen uptake from work rate is markedly greater on these tests compared with individualized tests.

Exercise Mode

Many modalities have been employed to stress the cardiovascular system, including steps, escalators, laddermills, and recently, drugs. Ideally, an exercise mode should be used that increases the work of the cardiopulmonary system to its highest level safely and within a reasonable period. Although isometric exercise has specific research applications, it causes inordinate increases in pressure and afterload rather than volume load on the ventricle. Dynamic exercise is most appropriate for exercise testing as it yields greater increases in cardiac output, oxygen delivery, and gas exchange. Large studies comparing the utility of pharmacologic stress to exercise testing are lacking.

The bicycle ergometer and the treadmill are the most commonly used dynamic exercise devices. The bicycle ergometer is usually cheaper, takes up less space, and makes less noise. Upper body motion is lessened, making blood pressure and ECG recordings easier. The workload administered by simple mechanically braked bicycle ergometers is not well calibrated and is dependent upon pedaling speed. Patients may slow down during exercise, thereby decreasing the workload administered. More expensive electronically braked bicycle ergometers maintain the workload at a specified level over a wide range of pedaling speeds. Bicycle ergometer work is usually expressed in kilogram meters per minute (kgm/min) or watts.

The treadmill is used most often for exercise testing in North America (12). It is usually more expensive than the cycle ergometer, it is relatively immobile, and it generally makes more noise. Newer models, however, are remarkably quiet. Researchers comparing treadmill and bicycle ergometer exercise tests have reported maximal oxygen uptake to be generally 10% to 20% higher (range 6% to 25%) (13,15,23,24) and maximal heart rate has been reported to be 5% to 20% higher on the treadmill. Not surprisingly, ST segment changes have been reported to be more frequent on the treadmill (24,25), and angina is elicited more frequently during treadmill testing compared with the cycle ergometer (15,24). Exercise-induced myocardial ischemia by thallium scintigraphy was recently reported to be much greater after treadmill testing versus that using a cycle ergometer (24). Although most of these differences have tended to be minor, if the functional limits of the patient and eliciting subjective or objective ischemia are important goals of the test, the treadmill may be preferable.

Handrails on the front and side of the treadmill are helpful so that patients can steady themselves. However, patients should be strongly discouraged from gripping the handrails. This decreases the work performed, decreases oxygen uptake, increases exercise time, and results in an overestimation of exercise capacity (26,27). Gripping the handrails also increases ECG muscle artifact. When not gripping the handrails, work can be estimated from treadmill speed and grade and expressed as predicted oxygen uptake or METs. Equations for predicting oxygen uptake from treadmill and cycle ergometer work rates are presented in appendix A.

Again, it is preferable to express exercise capacity as an MET value rather than as exercise time. This allows for comparison between different protocols. Also, there are many pitfalls to predicting exercise capacity on a treadmill or cycle ergometer, and MET values are usually overpredicted in patients with heart disease (15,16,21,28). The only accurate method of measuring work is ventilatory gas exchange analysis. (These techniques are described in chapters 3, 4, and 5.)

Patient Preparation

An important role of the physician supervising the test involves patient assessment before beginning. Exercise testing should be an extension of the history and physical examination. Contraindications to testing (Table 2.2) can be ruled out at this time (3). The referring physician should be contacted if the reason for the test is not clear. If there is doubt as to the purpose or safety of the test, it should not be performed at that time. Specific questioning should determine which medications are being taken, and potential electrolyte abnormalities should be considered. For routine testing, withdrawal of cardiac medicines is usually not recommended; the potential dangers of sudden withdrawal of beta-blocking agents have been well documented. If withdrawal is considered necessary for diagnostic testing, this process should be carefully supervised by a physician or nurse.

The patient should come to the laboratory appropriately dressed for exercise and be instructed not to eat, drink caffeinated beverages, or smoke at least three hours before the test. The adverse hemodynamic and symptomatic effects of food, caffeine, and tobacco consumption in close proximity to the exercise test among patients with heart disease have been described at length (29). Those

Table 2.2   Absolute and Relative Contraindications to Exercise Testing Outlined by the American Heart Association

Absolute	Relative*
Acute myocardial infarction or recent change in resting electrocardiogram	Less serious noncardiac disorder
Active unstable angina	Significant arterial or pulmonary hypertension
Serious cardiac arrhythmias	Tachyarrhythmias or bradyarrhythmias
Acute pericarditis	Moderate valvular or myocardial heart disease
Endocarditis	
Severe aortic stenosis	Drug effect or electrolyte abnormalities
Severe left ventricular dysfunction	Left main coronary obstruction or its equivalent
Acute pulmonary embolus or pulmonary infarction	Hypertrophic cardiomyopathy
Acute or serious noncardiac disorder	Psychiatric disease
Severe physical handicap or disability	

*Under certain circumstances and with appropriate precautions, relative contraindications can be superseded.

supervising the test should carefully explain the potential discomforts and risks to the patient. This explanation should include a demonstration of how to perform the test and how to end the test if the patient wishes to do so. There is sufficient legal precedent to recommend that all subjects sign an informed consent before undergoing an exercise test.

Although less emphasis has been placed on informed consent when testing apparently healthy individuals or athletes, the literature is replete with examples of legal case law arising from untoward responses in the exercise lab. In such individuals, diagnostic testing is of minimal value; the test is more commonly performed to assess fitness and efficacy of training. As such, the focus is commonly placed on gas exchange and lactate responses, running economy, endurance evaluations, and research. On rare occasions, initial screening of athletes raises questions regarding subclinical heart disease, and the exercise test is indicated as part of further workup. When routinely testing young, healthy individuals, it is generally not necessary to have a physician present (2). As with patients, the protocol and sequence of the test should be carefully explained. Contraindications to testing are the same for athletes as for the general population.

Heart Rate

Heart rate increases linearly with oxygen uptake during exercise. Of the two major components of cardiac output—heart rate and stroke volume—heart rate is responsible for most of the increase in cardiac output during exercise, particularly at higher levels. Thus, maximal heart rate achieved is a major determinant of exercise capacity (30,31). The inability to appropriately increase heart rate during exercise (**chronotropic incompetence**) has been associated with the presence of heart disease and a worse prognosis relative to patients who exhibit normal heart rate responses (32). Although maximal heart rate has been difficult to explain physiologically, it is affected by age, gender, health, type of exercise, body position, blood volume, and environment. Of these factors, age is the most important: there is an inverse relationship between maximal heart rate and age, with correlation coefficients in the order of −0.40. However, the scatter around the regression line is large, with standard deviations ranging from 10 to 15 beats/min. Thus, age-predicted maximal heart rate is a limited measurement for clinical purposes and should not be used as an endpoint for exercise testing.

Heart rate during exercise is also affected by the method of recording. Some of these methods have included arterial pulse oximetry, which is greatly affected by artifact, and cardiotachometers, which may either fail to trigger or inappropriately trigger on T-waves, artifact, or aberrant beats, thus yielding inaccurate results. Averaging heart rate over the last minute of exercise or in immediate recovery is common but inaccurate, since heart rate drops quickly in recovery and can climb steeply even in the final seconds of exercise. These problems are accentuated by patients with frequent dysrhythmias, and particularly among patients with atrial fibrillation. Atwood et al. (33) compared nine methods of sampling heart rate at rest and during exercise in normals and patients with chronic atrial fibrillation. These investigators concluded that the number of R-R intervals multiplied by 10 in a 6-sec rhythm strip represented a reasonable balance between convenience and precision for measuring heart rate during exercise, even in the presence of atrial fibrillation.

Arterial Blood Pressure

Arterial blood pressure reflects the increase in cardiac output and reduction in peripheral resistance that occur during exercise. Systolic pressure normally rises with increasing dynamic exercise while diastolic pressure remains roughly constant, yielding a modest rise in mean arterial pressure. Although many devices have been developed to automate the measurement of blood pressure during exercise, these devices lack validation, and it is preferable to take blood pressures manually. In a recent review of common errors in the indirect measurement of blood pressure, Bailey and Bauer (34) reported that roughly half the electronic or automated blood pressure devices tested at rest were found to have less than satisfactory accuracy and/or reliability. Naturally, exercise would exacerbate these problems.

An inadequate systolic blood pressure response to exercise (a rise that is less than 20 to 30 mmHg) may reflect left ventricular dysfunction, ischemia, or aortic outflow obstruction. If systolic blood pressure appears to be increasing sluggishly or decreasing, it should be taken again immediately. If a drop in systolic blood pressure of 10 to 20 mmHg or more occurs or if it drops below the value obtained standing before testing, the test should be stopped in patients with known heart disease or those who are exhibiting signs/symptoms of ischemia. The clinical significance of an abnormal blood pressure response to exercise ranges from modest (35,36) to severe, in which decreases in systolic blood pressure have been associated with ventricular fibrillation (37). Dubach et al. (38) have observed that systolic blood pressure must drop below the standing resting value to be prognostically valuable. Precise cut points and their significance are argued, but usually an increase in systolic blood pressure > 250 to 260 mmHg or an increase in diastolic blood pressure to 115 to 120 mmHg is an indication that the test should be stopped (2).

THE ELECTROCARDIOGRAM

Although the scope of exercise testing today includes a variety of techniques, such as echocardiographic, nuclear, gas exchange, nonexercise pharmacologic stress, and invasive methods, at the cornerstone of the exercise test clinically remains the concept that increasing myocardial oxygen demand in patients with cardiovascular disease causes changes in the electrocardiogram. Other available texts cover the diagnostic and prognostic applications of the exercise electrocardiogram in detail (39-42). Even when the focus of an exercise test is on one of these alternative techniques, patient safety considerations mandate a high-quality exercise electrocardiogram. The following sections discuss methodological considerations regarding skin preparation, lead systems, and computerization of the exercise electrocardiogram.

Among clinically referred patients or those with known heart disease, a resting 12-lead ECG should be obtained in both the supine and standing positions. In some patients, ECG shifts may occur from the supine to standing positions (particularly the appearance of inferior Q-waves). The physician should carefully review the resting tracings to rule out any contraindications to testing. The standing tracing is the baseline to which ECG changes during exercise are compared.

Lead Systems

Many lead systems and methods of placing electrodes have been used over the years. This situation has complicated making comparisons of the ST segment response to exercise. Many studies comparing the relative sensitivity of different lead systems were reported in the 1970s. The four major exercise electrocardiographic lead systems are the bipolar, the Mason-Likar 12-lead, a simulation of Wilson's central terminal, and the three-dimensional (orthogonal or nonorthogonal systems). Inconsistency is less of an issue today because all

ROUTINES TO KNOW:
PREPARING SKIN FOR EXERCISE TESTING

Because noise increases with the square of resistance, it is extremely important to lower the resistance at the skin-electrode interface and thereby improve the signal-to-noise ratio. An exercise test with an electrocardiographic signal that cannot be continuously monitored and accurately interpreted because of artifact is worthless and can even be dangerous. Preparing the skin properly often causes minor discomfort and skin irritation to the patient. The following list describes the standard procedure for skin preparation:

1. Shave the general areas for electrode placement.
2. Clean the areas with an alcohol-saturated gauze pad.
3. Mark the exact areas for electrode application with a felt-tip pen.
4. Before attaching the electrodes, remove the superficial layer of skin with fine-grain emery paper or steel wool.

commercially available systems employ 12-leads. While early studies used bipolar systems because of their simplicity, Mason and Likar were the first to attach electrodes to the base of the limbs during exercise (Figure 2.3) (43). Besides providing an exercise tracing with much less artifact, their modified placement showed no apparent differences in electrocardiographic configuration when compared with standard limb lead placement. However, this has been disputed by others who have found that the Mason-Likar placement causes amplitude changes and axis shifts when compared with standard placement (44-46). Since this could lead to diagnostic changes, it has been recommended that the modified exercise electrode placement not be used for recording a resting ECG. Differences between the standard ECG with the electrodes placed on the limbs and torso placement can be minimized by placing the arm electrodes as close to the shoulders as possible, attaching the leg electrodes below the umbilicus, and recording the resting ECG with the patient supine (44).

Although multiple lead systems are the standard today, the vast majority (perhaps greater than 90%) of ST segment changes will occur in the lateral precordial (chest) leads. Several investigators have reported that 10% to 20% of abnormal responses will be missed if 12-lead systems are not recorded (47,48).

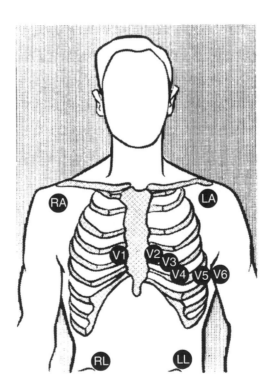

Figure 2.3 The Mason-Likar simulated 12-lead ECG electrode placement for exercise testing (43). Reprinted from Froelicher et al. 1993.

However, in subjects with normal resting ECGs and a low likelihood of coronary disease, recording more than the lateral leads is probably not useful. Miranda and associates (49) recently studied 178 males who had undergone both exercise testing and coronary angiography to evaluate the diagnostic value of ST segment depression occurring in the inferior leads. The superiority of the lateral leads versus the inferior leads was evident over multiple cut points, and ST depression isolated to lead II was unreliable. It remains to be demonstrated what the specificity of leads other than V_5 is, but these data give the impression that ST depression isolated to the inferior leads is frequently a **false positive response**.

Computerization

Equipment manufacturers today rely heavily on computers for signal processing. Most systems now use analogue and digital techniques to average ECG signals and remove noise. Table 2.3 summarizes the results of studies evaluating the **sensitivity** and **specificity** of the visual and computerized exercise ECG compared with thallium scintigraphy. These data suggest that the computer has indeed led to an improvement in test sensitivity. However, a need exists for consumer awareness in these areas, since most manufacturers do not specify how the use of such procedures modifies the ECG. Signal averaging can actually distort the ECG signal. These techniques are attractive because they can produce a clean tracing in spite of poor skin preparation. However, the common expression used by computer scientists, ''garbage in, garbage out,'' has never been more applicable than to the ECG. The clean-looking ECG signal produced may not be a true representation of the actual waveform and may in fact be misleading. Also, the instruments that measure computer ST segments are not totally reliable, since they are based on algorithms designed by humans and are inherently imperfect. While it may be seductive to employ the latest computer measurement or score to all patients, the wisdom of applying any given score to all populations must be questioned (50-52). It is important to note that although these new technologies

Table 2.3   Summary of Angiographic Studies Using Computerized Exercise Electrocardiography Versus Visual ECG Analysis, Thallium, and Radionuclide Ventriculography (RNV) for the Diagnosis of Coronary Artery Disease

	Computer ECG $n = 10$	Visual ECG $n = 33$	Thallium $n = 16$	RNV $n = 7$
Sensitivity	80%	66%	76%	93%
Specificity	91%	84%	89%	79%

n = number of reported studies.

Reprinted from Froelicher, Myers, Follansbee, and Labovitz 1993.

have facilitated precision, convenience, and perhaps test accuracy, they should be used with discretion. The averages should be used as a supplement; one should first view the raw ECG data for distortion, make measurements over at least three consecutive, consistent complexes, and then check the averages for agreement. The averages can be used as a summary of the results if they agree with the raw data. Skin preparation is critical to obtaining reliable raw or averaged signals.

Assessing Maximal Effort

Although many efforts have been made to objectify maximal effort, such as age-predicted maximal heart rate, a plateau in oxygen uptake, exceeding the **ventilatory threshold (VT)**, or a **respiratory exchange ratio (RER)** greater than unity, all have considerable measurement error and intersubject variability (16,32,53-55). This is true despite the presence or absence of disease. The 95% confidence limits for maximal heart rate based on age, for example, range nearly 50 beats/min; therefore, this endpoint is maximal for some and submaximal for others (32). The classic index of one's cardiopulmonary limits, a plateau in oxygen uptake, is not observed in many patients, is poorly reproducible, and has been confused by many criteria applied (53-55). (This issue is discussed in more detail in chapter 4.) Though subjective, the Borg perceived exertion scale is helpful for assessing exercise effort (Figure 2.4) (56). Good judgment by the physician remains the most effective criteria for ending exercise.

6	No exertion at all
7	
8	Extremely light
9	Very light
10	
11	Light
12	
13	Somewhat hard
14	
15	Hard
16	
17	Very hard
18	
19	Extremely hard
20	Maximal exertion

Figure 2.4   The Borg 6-20 perceived exertion scale (56). Reprinted from Borg 1985.

Clinical indications for stopping an exercise test are listed in Table 2.4 (2). Most problems can be avoided by having an experienced physician, nurse, or exercise physiologist standing next to the patient, measuring blood pressure, and assessing patient appearance during the test. The exercise technician should operate the recorder and treadmill, take appropriate tracings, enter data on a form, and alert the physician to any abnormalities that may appear on the monitor scope. If the patient's appearance is worrisome, systolic blood pressure plateaus or drops, marked electrocardiographic changes occur, chest pain becomes worse than the patient's usual pain, or the patient wants to stop the test for any reason, the test should be stopped, even at apparent submaximal levels. A great deal of effort has been directed toward the assessment of chest pain during exercise testing (29). Our preference has been to use a 1-4 scaling system (Figure 2.5), in which the test is terminated at a rating of 3, indicating the patient has reached a "moderately severe" level of chest discomfort, or a point at which the patient would stop and rest and/or take a sublingual nitroglycerin pill during normal daily activities. This scale is particularly useful when using gas exchange techniques because chest pain sensations can be expressed nonverbally with simple hand signals. Usually, a symptom-limited maximal test is preferred, but it is usually advisable to stop if 0.2 mm of ST segment elevation occurs or if 0.2 mm flat or downsloping ST depression occurs (2,3).

Table 2.4 Indications for Stopping an Exercise Test

1. Progressive angina (stop at 3+ level or earlier on a scale of 1+ to 4+)
2. Ventricular tachycardia
3. Any significant drop (20 mmHg) of systolic blood pressure
4. Lightheadedness, confusion, ataxia, pallor, cyanosis, nausea, or signs of severe peripheral circulatory insufficiency
5. > 2 mm horizontal or downsloping ST depression or elevation (in the absence of other indicators of ischemia)
6. Onset of second- or third-degree A-V block
7. Increasing ventricular ectopy, multiform PVCs, or R on T PVCs
8. Excessive rise in blood pressure: systolic pressure > 250 mmHg; diastolic pressure > 120 mmHg
9. Chronotropic impairment
10. Sustained supraventricular tachycardia
11. Exercise-induced left bundle branch block
12. Subject asks to stop
13. Failure of the monitoring system

AV = atrioventricular; PVCs = premature ventricular contractions.

Reprinted from American College of Sports Medicine 1995.

Levels of Chest Discomfort

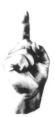

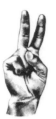

1 ONSET OF DISCOMFORT
You notice chest sensation.

2 MODERATE DISCOMFORT
You feel the pain increasing.

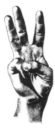

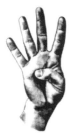

3 MODERATELY SEVERE
The discomfort would cause
you to rest or take nitroglycerin.

4 SEVERE DISCOMFORT

Figure 2.5 Rating scale for exertional chest discomfort. The scale is particularly useful when using gas exchange techniques, as chest discomfort can be expressed non-verbally using hand signals. A rating of three is the appropriate endpoint. Reprinted from Myers et al. 1994.

Postexercise Period

Some debate exists as to whether the patient should immediately be placed supine or allowed a cooldown period (slow walking or light pedaling) after the exercise test. Diagnostic sensitivity of the test appears to be improved if patients are placed supine during the postexercise period. Because the increase in venous return and thus ventricular volume in the supine position boosts myocardial oxygen demand, it has been suggested that a cooldown walk can delay or eliminate the appearance of ST segment depression. Data from Lachterman et al. (57) and Gutman et al. (58) suggest that the supine position may enhance ST segment abnormalities in recovery. Others have suggested that a cooldown walk can minimize the chances for dysrhythmic events in this high-risk time when catecholamines are elevated (5). The supine position postexercise is not so important when the test is not being performed for diagnostic purposes (i.e., for research purposes or fitness evaluations). We use cooldown periods in our research lab (where testing is not performed for diagnostic reasons), but in our clinical laboratory (where diagnostic testing is performed) nearly all patients are placed in the supine position immediately. For patients who exhibit ominous arrhythmias, a cooldown walk may be appropriate. When this is the case, it may be preferable to walk slowly (1.0 to 1.5 mph) or continue cycling against zero or minimal resistance (0 to 25 watts) for several minutes following the test. Monitoring should continue for at least 6 to 8 min after exercise or until both the ECG and blood pressure are stable. An abnormal response occurring only in the recovery period is not unusual and may significantly improve test sensitivity (57).

SUMMARY

Appropriate attention to proper methodology is essential to optimize the information yield from the exercise test. Standards developed by major organizations (American Heart Association, American College of Cardiology, American College of Sports Medicine, American College of Physicians) that address methods, interpretation, personnel, and safety issues have been helpful in bringing uniformity to the exercise laboratory. These standards include not only guidelines concerning methodology but also physician and technician requirements, competency, and certification.

The exercise protocol should be progressive with equal increments in work rate whenever possible. Smaller, equivalent, and more frequent work increments are preferable to larger, uneven increments because they yield a more accurate estimate of exercise capacity. Recent studies on optimizing the exercise test have suggested that the test should be individualized to yield a duration ranging between 8 and 12 min. Ramp testing facilitates many of the recent recommendations concerning optimizing the exercise test.

Exercise capacity should not be reported in total exercise time but rather the oxygen uptake or MET equivalent of the workload achieved. This permits comparison of the results between exercise protocols. Testing endpoints should be based on published guidelines and clinical judgment. Target heart rates based on age should not be used because the relationship between maximal heart rate and age is poor, and there is a wide scatter around the different published regression lines.

The cornerstone of the exercise test clinically remains the electrocardiographic response. Computers have engendered a new era in exercise testing methodology, but they have also brought new problems. Despite years of study, the optimal computer criteria for myocardial ischemia continues to be disputed. In addition to the measurements used, the ECG response to exercise is strongly influenced by patient preparation, the lead system employed, medications, and adequacy of patient effort. Studies have shown that using leads in addition to V_5 will increase test sensitivity slightly; however, the specificity is decreased. Recent studies have also shown that ST segment changes isolated to the inferior leads are often false positive responses. The recovery period appears to be extremely important, and ST changes isolated in the recovery period should not be discarded.

REFERENCES

1. American Association of Cardiovascular and Pulmonary Rehabilitation. 1995. Guidelines for Cardiac Rehabilitation Programs, 2d ed. Champaign, IL: Human Kinetics.
2. American College of Sports Medicine. 1995. Guidelines for Exercise Testing and Exercise Prescription, 5th ed. Philadelphia: Lea and Febiger.
3. Fletcher GF, Froelicher VF, Hartley LH, Haskell WL, Pollock ML. 1995. Exercise standards: A statement for health professionals from the American Heart Association. Circulation 91: 580-615.
4. Schlant R, Friesinger GC, Leonard JJ. 1987. Clinical competence in exercise testing. A statement for physicians from the ACP/ACC/AHA task force on clinical privileges in cardiology. Ann Intern Med 107: 588-589.
5. Gibbons L, Blair SN, Kohl HW, Cooper K. 1989. The safety of maximal exercise testing. Circulation 80: 846-852.
6. Rochmis P, Blackburn H. 1971. Exercise tests: A survey of procedures, safety, and litigation experience in approximately 170,000 tests. J Am Med Assoc 217: 1061.
7. Franklin B, Dressendorfer R, Hollingsworth V, Buchal M, Gordon S, Timms G. 1990. Safety of exercise testing by non-physician health care providers: Twelve-year experience. Circulation 82 (suppl III): III-135.
8. Balke B, Ware R. 1959. An experimental study of physical fitness of Air Force personnel. U.S. Armed Forces Med J 10: 675-688.
9. Åstrand PO, Rodahl K. 1986. Textbook of Work Physiology, 331-365. New York: McGraw-Hill.
10. Bruce RA. 1971. Exercise testing of patients with coronary heart disease. Ann Clin Res 3: 323-330.
11. Ellestad MH, Allen W, Wan MCK, Kemp G. 1969. Maximal treadmill stress testing for cardiovascular evaluation. Circulation 39: 517-522.
12. Stuart RJ, Ellestad MH. 1980. National survey of exercise stress testing facilities. Chest 77: 94-97.
13. Buchfuhrer MJ, Hansen JE, Robinson TE, Sue DY, Wasserman K, Whipp BJ. 1983. Optimizing the exercise protocol for cardiopulmonary assessment. J Appl Physiol 55: 1558-1564.
14. Haskell W, Savin W, Oldridge N, DeBusk R. 1982. Factors influencing estimated oxygen uptake during exercise testing soon after myocardial infarction. Am J Cardiol 50: 299-304.
15. Myers J, Buchanan N, Walsh D, Kraemer M, McAuley P, Hamilton-Wessler M, Froelicher VF. 1991. Comparison of the ramp versus standard exercise protocols. J Am Coll Cardiol 17: 1334-1342.
16. Myers J, Froelicher VF. 1990. Optimizing the exercise test for pharmacological investigations. Circulation 82: 1839-1846.
17. Myers J, Buchanan N, Smith D, Neutel J, Bowes E, Walsh D, Froelicher VF. 1992. Individualized ramp treadmill: Observations on a new protocol. Chest 101: 2305-2415.

18. Redwood DR, Rosing DR, Goldstein RE, Beiser GD, Epstein SE. 1971. Importance of the design of an exercise protocol in the evaluation of patients with angina pectoris. Circulation 43: 618-628.
19. Webster MWI, Sharpe DN. 1989. Exercise testing in angina pectoris: The importance of protocol design in clinical trials. Am Heart J 117: 505 508.
20. Tamesis B, Stelken A, Byers S, Shaw L, Younis L, Miller D, Chaitman B. 1993. Comparison of the asymptomatic cardiac ischemia pilot and modified asymptomatic cardiac ischemia pilot versus Bruce and Cornell exercise protocols. Am J Cardiol 72: 715-720.
21. Sullivan M, McKirnan MD. 1984. Errors in predicting functional capacity for postmyocardial infarction patients using a modified Bruce protocol. Am Heart J 107: 486-491.
22. Panza J, Quyyumi AA, Diodati JG, Callaham TS, Epstein SE. 1991. Prediction of the frequency and duration of ambulatory myocardial ischemia in patients with stable coronary artery disease by determination of the ischemic threshold from exercise testing: Importance of the exercise protocol. J Am Coll Cardiol 17: 657-663.
23. Hermanson L, Saltin B. 1969. Oxygen uptake during maximal treadmill and bicycle exercise. J Appl Physiol 26: 31-37.
24. Hambrecht R, Schuler GC, Muth T, Grunze MF, Marfinger CT, Niebauer J, Methfessel SM, Kubler W. 1992. Greater diagnostic sensitivity of treadmill versus cycle exercise testing of asymptomatic men with coronary artery disease. Am J Cardiol 70: 141-146.
25. Wicks JR, Sutton JR, Oldridge NB, Jones NL. 1978. Comparison of the electrocardiographic changes induced by maximum exercise testing with treadmill and cycle ergometer. Circulation 57: 1066-1069.
26. Von Duvillard SP, Pivirotto JM. 1991. The effect of front handrail and nonhandrail support on treadmill exercise in healthy women. J Cardiopulmonary Rehabil 11: 164-168.
27. Zeimetz GA, McNeill JF, Hall JR, Moss RF. 1985. Quantifiable changes in oxygen uptake, heart rate, and time to target heart rate when hand support is allowed during treadmill exercise. J Cardiopulmonary Rehabil 5: 525-530.
28. Roberts JM, Sullivan M, Froelicher VF, Genter F, Myers J. 1984. Predicting oxygen uptake from treadmill testing in normal subjects and coronary artery disease patients. Am Heart J 108: 1454-1460.
29. Myers J, Froelicher VF. 1995. Optimizing the exercise test for pharmacologic interventions in patients with angina pectoris. In D Ardissino, S Savonitto, and LH Opie, eds. Drug Evaluation in Angina Pectoris, 41-52. Boston: Kluwer Academic.
30. McKirnan MD, Sullivan M, Jensen D, Froelicher VF. 1984. Treadmill performance and cardiac function in selected patients with coronary heart disease. J Am Coll Cardiol 3: 253-261.
31. Myers J, Froelicher VF. 1985. Hemodynamic determinants of exercise capacity in chronic heart failure. Ann Intern Med 115: 377-386.

32. Hammond K, Froelicher VF. Normal and abnormal heart rate responses to exercise. Prog Cardiovasc Dis 27: 271-296.
33. Atwood JE, Myers J, Sandhu S, Lachterman B, Friis R, Oshita A, Forbes S, Walsh D, Froelicher VF. 1989. Optimal sampling interval to estimate heart rate at rest and during exercise in atrial fibrillation. Am J Cardiol 63: 45-48.
34. Bailey RH, Bauer JH. 1993. A review of common errors in the indirect measurement of blood pressure. Arch Intern Med 153: 2741-2748.
35. Mazzotta G, Scopinaro G, Falcidieno M, Claudiani F, DeCaro E, Bonow RO, Vecchio C. 1987. Significance of abnormal blood pressure response during exercise-induced myocardial dysfunction after recent acute myocardial infarction. Am J Cardiol 59: 1256-1260.
36. Levites R, Baker T, Anderson GJ. 1978. The significance of hypotension developing during treadmill exercise testing. Am Heart J 95: 747-753.
37. Irving JB, Bruce RA. 1977. Exertional hypotension and postexertional ventricular fibrillation in stress testing. Am J Cardiol 39: 849-851.
38. Dubach P, Froelicher VF, Klein J, Oakes D, Grover-McKay M, Friis R. 1989. Exercise-induced hypotension in a male population: Criteria, causes, and prognosis. Circulation 78: 1380-1387.
39. Ellestad MH. 1986. Stress Testing: Principles and Practice. Philadelphia: FA Davis.
40. Chung EK. 1983. Exercise Electrocardiography: Practical Approach. Baltimore: Williams and Wilkins.
41. Froelicher VF, Myers J, Follansbee WP, Labovitz AJ. 1993. Exercise and the Heart, 3d ed. St. Louis: Mosby-Year Book.
42. Froelicher VF. 1994. Manual of Exercise Testing, 2d ed. St. Louis: Mosby-Year Book.
43. Mason RE, Likar I. 1966. A new system of multiple-lead exercise electrocardiography. Am Heart J 71: 196-205.
44. Gamble P, McManus H, Jensen D, Froelicher VF. 1984. A comparison of the standard 12-lead electrocardiogram to exercise electrode placements. Chest 85: 616-622.
45. Kleiner JP, Nelson WP, Boland MJ. 1978. The 12-lead electrocardiogram in exercise testing. Arch Intern Med 138: 1572-1573.
46. Rautaharju PM, Prineas RJ, Crow RS, Seale D, Furberg C. 1980. The effect of modified limb positions on electrocardiographic wave amplitudes. J Electrocardiol 13: 109-113.
47. Robertson D, Kostuk WJ, Ajuja SP. 1976. The localization of coronary artery stenoses by 12-lead ECG response to graded exercise test: Support for intercoronary steal. Am Heart J 91: 437.
48. Tucker SC, Kemp VE, Holland WE, et al. 1976. Multiple lead ECG submaximal treadmill exercise tests in angiographically documented coronary heart disease. Angiology 27: 149.
49. Miranda CP, Liu J, Kadar A, Janosi A, Froning J, Lehmann KG, Froelicher VF. 1992. Usefulness of exercise-induced ST-segment depression in the

inferior leads during exercise testing as a marker for coronary artery disease. Am J Cardiol 69: 303-307.

50. Ribisl PM, Liu J, Mousa I, Herbert WG, Miranda CP, Froning JN, Froelicher VF. 1993. Comparison of computer ST criteria for diagnosis of severe coronary artery disease. Am J Cardiol 71: 546-551.

51. Milliken JA, Abdollah H, Burggraf GW. 1990. False-positive treadmill exercise tests due to computer signal averaging. Am J Cardiol 65: 946-948.

52. Lachterman B, Lehmann KG, Detrano R, Neutel J, Froelicher VF. 1990. Comparison of ST segment/heart rate index to standard ST criteria for analysis of exercise electrocardiogram. Circulation 82: 44-50.

53. Myers J, Walsh D, Buchanan N, Froelicher VF. 1989. Can maximal cardiopulmonary capacity be recognized by a plateau in oxygen uptake? Chest 96: 1312-1316.

54. Myers J, Walsh D, Sullivan M, Froelicher VF. 1990. Effect of sampling on variability and plateau in oxygen uptake. J Appl Physiol 68 (1): 404-410.

55. Stachenfeld NS, Eskenazi M, Gleim GW, Coplan NL, Nicholas JA. 1992. Predictive accuracy of criteria used to assess maximal oxygen consumption. Am Heart J 123: 922.

56. Borg G. 1985. An Introduction to Borg's RPE-Scale. Ithaca, NY: Mouvement Publications.

57. Lachterman B, Lehmann KG, Abrahamson D, Froelicher VF. 1990. ''Recovery only'' ST segment depression and the predictive accuracy of the exercise test. Ann Intern Med 112: 11-16.

58. Gutman RA, Alexander ER, Li YB, Chiang BN. 1970. Delay of ST depression after maximal exercise by walking for two minutes. Circulation 42: 229-233.

59. Whipp BJ, Davis JA, Torres F, Wasserman, K. 1981. A test to determine parameters of aerobic function during exercise. J Appl Physiol 50: 217 221.

CHAPTER

3

INSTRUMENTATION: EQUIPMENT, CALCULATIONS, AND VALIDATION

*T*he measurement of cardiopulmonary gas exchange variables brings an added dimension to the exercise test. When done properly, gas exchange techniques enhance precision and provide a considerable increase in information concerning the patient's cardiopulmonary function. The use of these techniques, however, requires added attention to detail and a working knowledge of the equipment and basic gas exchange physiology. This working knowledge is particularly important today because advances in technology have greatly automated the process of acquiring gas exchange data. It is easy to be seduced by the speed and convenience, for example, of autocalibration or autothreshold determination programs and the many versions of computerized data output available without paying proper attention to instrumentation and the calibration process. These points will be emphasized repeatedly throughout the remainder of the text, and the last section of this chapter has been devoted strictly to data validation and quality control.

The purpose of this chapter is to describe the instrumentation and theory behind the measurement of gas exchange variables. The issues discussed include the calculation of oxygen uptake, the systems available to measure the concentrations of oxygen and carbon dioxide, methods used to acquire ventilation, how the data are sampled and the conditions under which they are expressed, quality control, system validation and calibration, and the theory and measurements used to determine cardiac output noninvasively from gas exchange data.

CALCULATION OF OXYGEN UPTAKE

In its simplest terms, the determination of oxygen uptake requires the ability to measure three variables:

- The fraction of oxygen in the expired air
- The fraction of carbon dioxide in the expired air
- The volume of the inspired or expired air

The volume of expired air is commonly collected with the use of a non-rebreathing valve, as illustrated in Figure 3.1. A sample line connected to the valve apparatus

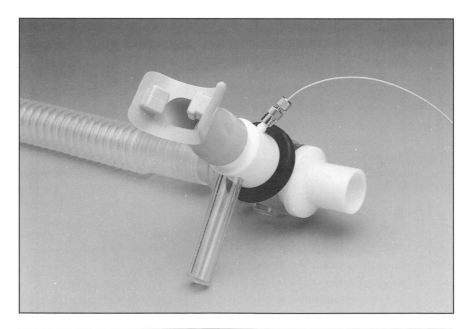

Figure 3.1 A one-way, T-shaped non-rebreathing valve with mouthpiece and saliva trap (manufactured by Hans Rudolph).

draws a continuous sample of expired air to measure the fractions of oxygen and carbon dioxide. Oxygen uptake can be described as simply the product of ventilation ($\dot{V}_E$) in a given interval and the fraction of oxygen in that ventilation that has been consumed by the working muscle:

$$\dot{V}O_2 \text{ ml/min (STPD)} = \dot{V}_E \times (F_IO_2 - F_EO_2),$$

where F_IO_2 is the fraction of inspired oxygen and F_EO_2 is the fraction of expired oxygen. F_IO_2 is equal to 20.93% at sea level and 0% humidity, and ventilation is converted to standard temperature and pressure, dry (STPD). $F_IO_2 - F_EO_2$ represents the amount of oxygen consumed by the working muscle for a given sample, sometimes called "**true O_2**." This difference in the concentration of oxygen in the ambient and exhaled air is measured using a metabolic system containing an oxygen analyzer. This process is illustrated in Figure 3.2.

For the sake of explanation, the above equation is oversimplified, as it assumes that expired air is dry and that the inspired and expired volumes are not different. Because this is generally not the case (inspired and expired volumes are similar only when the respiratory exchange ratio equals one), several additional calculations are necessary to accurately determine oxygen uptake. First, the sample of inspired air must be dried, or the humidity in the room must be measured and F_IO_2 adjusted accordingly. Second, because oxygen uptake is the difference between the fraction of oxygen in the inspired and expired ventilation, both inspired and expired ventilation must be known precisely. Ventilatory volume is frequently measured only from the expired air. Inspired volume, however, can be determined from the expired volume and the fractions of oxygen and carbon dioxide. This is possible because nitrogen (N_2) and other inert gases do not affect

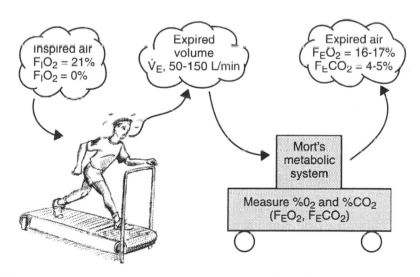

Figure 3.2 Method of obtaining oxygen uptake by measuring the volume and concentration of exhaled air.

the body's gas exchange processes. In other words, the amount of N_2 inspired is equal to the amount of N_2 expired. We need only concern ourselves with differences in the concentrations of O_2 and CO_2 between the inspired and expired air. The concentrations of N_2, CO_2, and O_2 in the inspired air (when dry) are known to approximate 0.7904, 0, and 0.2093, respectively. The fraction of inert gases in the expired air (F_EN_2) is

$$F_EN_2 = 1 - F_EO_2 - F_ECO_2$$

Thus, inspiratory volume ($\dot{V}_I$) can be expressed as the difference between the fraction of inert gases in the expired air and the fraction of inert gases in the atmosphere:

$$\dot{V}_I = \frac{[\dot{V}_E \times (1 - F_EO_2 - F_ECO_2)]}{0.7904}$$

The equation for oxygen uptake then becomes

$$\dot{V}O_2 \text{ L/min STPD} = \frac{(1 - F_EO_2 - F_ECO_2)}{0.7904} \times (F_IO_2 - F_EO2) \times \dot{V}_E \text{ L/min STPD}$$

The fraction of oxygen in the ambient air (F_IO_2) changes with the relative humidity and temperature. The relationship between ambient oxygen and relative humidity is inverse, and ambient oxygen is slightly lower as temperature increases (Figure 3.3). Some systems take the effects of humidity and temperature into account and measure the F_IO_2 directly. Some systems dry the sample and assume

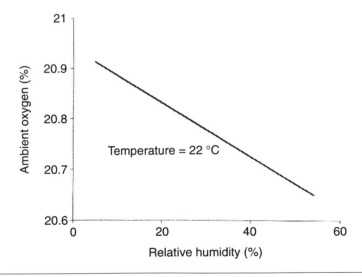

Figure 3.3 The relationship between ambient oxygen, expressed as a percentage, and relative humidity at a temperature of 22 °C. The slope of this relationship steepens slightly as temperature increases and flattens as temperature decreases.

an F_IO_2 of 20.93%, while others standardize the system with a calibration gas containing approximately 21% O_2.

COLLECTION OF EXPIRED VENTILATION

The measurement of ventilation during exercise requires that the patient's nose and mouth be sealed tightly with a clip and a mouthpiece. The non-rebreathing valve illustrated in Figure 3.1 is a one-way valve; that is, differences in pressure occurring with inhalation and exhalation open and close the valves (often in the form of a rubber diaphragm) so that air flows in one direction and inspired and expired air do not mix. The three ports on the valve are for inspired air, expired air, and the patient, respectively. All breathing valves have a "dead space," a volume of air that fills the valve apparatus and does not participate in gas exchange. A balance exists between the dead space volume and the valve's resistance: the smaller the dead space, the higher the resistance. Both high dead space and high resistance are undesirable, and most exercise testing is performed using a valve with a dead space less than 100 ml. Although face masks are available that cover the nose and mouth (making speaking possible), care must be taken so that leaking does not occur at high ventilation rates. Newer face masks are less apt to leak, have a small dead space (40 ml), and are more comfortable than older masks, since they permit the subject to swallow or speak (Figure 3.4). Speaking should be discouraged, however, because it can interfere with the metabolic system's ability to define breaths.

According to the equation for oxygen uptake on p. 62, expired gas analysis requires that the gases be analyzed for total volume as well as oxygen and carbon dioxide content. Accurate measurement requires that water content be quantified and adjustments made for standard pressure and temperature (thus, the correction for STPD); more on this in a moment. As originally performed, expired gases were collected in a Tissot. This device was an inverted metal cylinder suspended in a large container filled with water. Filling the inner cylinder with expired air caused it to rise in the water, and ventilation was measured as the degree of displacement of the cylinder. Other methods of measuring air volume required Douglas bags or weather balloons, using a turret that rotated from one bag to the next at given time intervals. These methods required a great deal of technician time and limited precision because sampling was dictated by the size of the collection bags and slowly responding analyzers. Because of the many recent advances in gas analysis systems, these methods are virtually obsolete in the laboratory setting. However, collection bag methods remain the only practical technique for measuring oxygen uptake during athletic events or in other field settings.

Collection bag systems for measuring gas volumes evolved into "mixing chamber" systems in which a given interval of exhaled air is briefly trapped in a collection chamber. This automates the process and allows the fractions of oxygen and carbon dioxide to be mixed completely, with the help of baffles

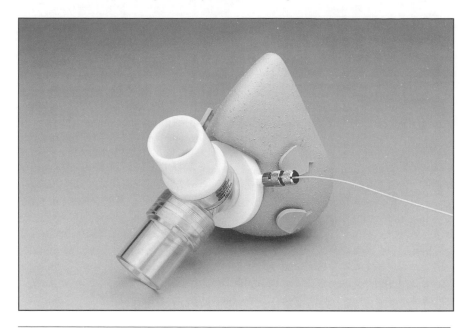

Figure 3.4   Face mask with two-way non-rebreathing valve (manufactured by Hans Rudolph).

inside the chamber. The sample is then pumped to a flow meter and gas analyzer. The mixing chamber method has numerous advantages over the collection bag technique, including the fact that it is less cumbersome and requires less technician time, and the patient responses are obtained more rapidly. However, mixing chambers still require certain mixing, equilibration, and ''wash out'' periods that limit the frequency with which data may be sampled.

Today, gas analysis is commonly performed ''on-line.'' Various types of flow meters are used including mass transducers, Fleisch **pneumotachometers**, hot-wire devices, or small propellers and turbines. These rapidly responding systems permit the measurement of gas exchange data on a breath-by-breath basis. With these systems, the patient's responses are available immediately, and with the help of a computer, rapid computations can be made and displayed continuously during the test.

- *Pneumotachometers* measure reductions in pressure caused by airflow through a tube or series of wire screens. The relationship between flow and a drop in pressure is stated by **Bernoulli's law** (flow is proportional to the square root of the pressure difference), and this permits the measurement of ventilation using a pneumotachometer.
- A *turbine* volume transducer uses a small impeller to measure bidirectional flow at the mouth. The impeller is spun in proportion to the rate of airflow.
- A *hot-wire* device, or *anemometer*, consists of a narrow tube with a heated wire on the inside. As air flows through the tube, it cools the wire. The

volume of airflow is proportional to the amount of electricity required to reheat the wire.

Among the problems with these devices is the difficulty in measuring ventilatory volume directly from a rapidly breathing individual. The phasic nature of breathing affects these devices. It has been suggested that most commercial devices which measure flow directly from a patient are not as accurate as "off-line" methods. However, many technological advances have occurred in this area in recent years, and these systems are now the norm commercially. There remains the need, though, to perform validation studies on these newer devices.

Three manufacturers have recently developed small, lightweight, disposable pneumotachometers that measure flow volume at the mouth (Figure 3.5). These clever devices obviate the need for headgear, the valve apparatus, and collection tubes, which can often be cumbersome. As inexpensive disposable devices, these systems also reduce the risk of contamination. Flow is determined as a difference in pressure between the front and back of a strut positioned in the center of the pneumotachometer. A schematic showing a breath-by-breath system including a disposable pneumotach, rapidly responding analyzers, and a microprocessor is presented in Figure 3.6. The three relevant breath-by-breath signals (flow, CO_2, and O_2) are aligned based on the response time and phase delay of the instruments in order to quantify the gas exchange data. A listing of the various manufacturers of gas exchange equipment is presented in appendix B.

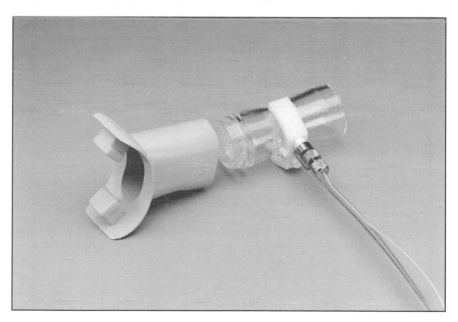

Figure 3.5 Disposable pneumotach developed by the Medical Graphics Corporation. Ventilatory volume is measured as a difference in pressure between the front and back of a strut positioned in the center.

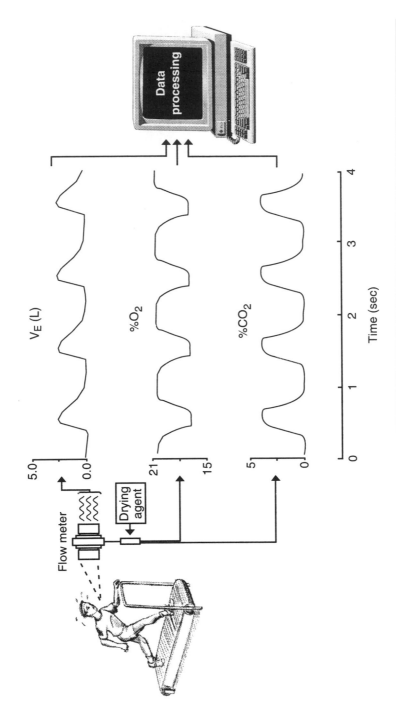

Figure 3.6 Schematic of an automated breath-by-breath system with the three electronic signals aligned to generate gas exchange data.

GAS ANALYZERS

The development of rapidly responding, computer-assisted gas analyzers is relatively recent. Early gas analysis systems consisted mainly of Haldane and Scholander methods, which were so cumbersome as to make them impractical in the exercise laboratory. The two types of oxygen analyzers commonly used today are the *paramagnetic* and *electrochemical*. These oxygen analyzers actually measure partial pressures; the gas is expressed as a percentage by taking the ratio of the partial pressure of oxygen to the barometric pressure.

Electrochemical analyzers are most often used by the automated systems available today. These systems commonly use a zirconium oxide cell heated to extreme temperatures. Differences in the partial pressure of oxygen on either side of the cell's semipermeable membrane (i.e., room air versus inside the sensor) generate a current proportional to the difference. The paramagnetic analyzer measures the change in a magnetic field caused by changes in the concentration of oxygen. This type of system is frequently used for portable O_2 analysis, but its response time is slow, and it is not often used for metabolic exercise systems.

Carbon dioxide is generally measured with an *infrared* analyzer. This is based on the idea that carbon dioxide absorbs energy from a specific portion of the infrared spectrum. Infrared light passes through a cell containing a given amount of carbon dioxide, and the volume of light transmitted is compared with a known constant value. The difference is proportional to the partial pressure of carbon dioxide in the sample. Infrared carbon dioxide analyzers have been well validated, have very fast response times, and are used in virtually all the commercially available metabolic systems.

CORRECTION OF GAS VOLUMES
TO STANDARD CONDITIONS

Generally, metabolic systems measure ventilatory volume under conditions of atmospheric temperature and pressure, saturated with water vapor (**ATPS**). That is, the system receives air from the patient that is saturated with water vapor under variable (ambient) conditions of temperature and pressure. An important distinction that must be made is that between a gas volume designated ATPS and those designated body temperature and pressure, saturated (BTPS), or standard temperature and pressure, dry (STPD). $\dot{V}O_2$ and $\dot{V}CO_2$ measurements need to be expressed under STPD conditions to make them proportional to gas exchanged in moles (an expression that incorporates both the absolute and molecular weight of a gas). The conventional standard conditions are a temperature of 0°C, a pressure of 760 mmHg, and a completely dry gas. Generally, gas exchange variables pertaining to volumes within the lung are expressed as BTPS, while those involving the exchange of gas between the lung and the bloodstream are expressed as STPD. Therefore, $\dot{V}_E$ is usually expressed in BTPS, whereas $\dot{V}O_2$ and $\dot{V}CO_2$ are expressed in STPD.

These differences are critical since water vapor can greatly influence the data. The concentration of the water molecules in a gas sample also varies with both the temperature and the barometric pressure. Thus, it is important that the system take into account each variable and that the data be reported in a fashion consistent with convention. One expression of ventilatory volume can be converted to another through some simple equations. Ventilation expressed as BTPS can be converted to ATPS by the following:

$$V_E \text{ (BTPS)} = V_E \text{ (ATPS)} \times \frac{Pb - P_{atm} (H_2O)}{Pb - 47 \text{ mmHg}} \times \frac{310}{273 + Ta} ,$$

where Pb is the barometric pressure, Ta is ambient temperature, and Pa (H_2O) is the water vapor pressure.

When the system uses **inspired ventilation (V_I)** rather than V_E to measure volume, V_I is an atmospheric condition (ATPS), and this conversion applies similarly.

Ventilation expressed as STPD can be converted to ATPS by the following:

$$V_E \text{ (STPD)} = V_E \text{ (ATPS)} \times \frac{Pb - P_{atm} (H_2O)}{760 \text{ mmHg}} \times \frac{273}{273 + Ta}$$

Conversion factors to change volumes measured under ATPS conditions to BTPS and STPD conditions at given temperature and water vapor pressures are available in tabular form.

GAS EXCHANGE DATA SAMPLING

Not long ago, gas exchange analysis was an awkward process that required the user to fill and empty ventilation bags at precise intervals. Sampling was limited to each minute, and the process was subject to a great deal of error. The recent availability of rapidly responding gas analyzers has provided the user with a choice as to how to sample the data on-line. This technology has certainly facilitated precision and convenience, but has led to confusion regarding data sampling. For example, differences in sampling (i.e., breath by breath, 30 sec, 60 sec, or "running" breath averaging) can greatly affect precision and variability in measuring oxygen uptake. Figure 3.7 illustrates the standard deviations of various oxygen uptake samples during steady-state exercise in 10 subjects (1). Not surprisingly, the variability in oxygen uptake is considerably greater as the sampling interval shortens (e.g., 4.5 ml/kg/min for breath-by-breath versus 0.8 ml/kg/min for 60-sec samples). Thus, a given value for oxygen uptake carries an inherent variability, and this variability depends on the sampling interval. Shorter sampling intervals increase resolution, making it possible to assess precise periods for certain applications, but also increase the variability.

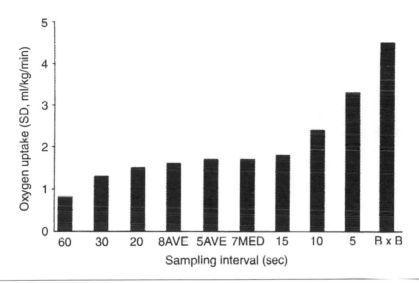

Figure 3.7 Variability in oxygen uptake expressed by the standard deviation for different sampling intervals during 5 min of steady-state exercise. 8AVE and 5AVE are "moving" breath averages, 7MED is the median of seven breaths, B × B is breath by breath. Reprinted from Myers et al. 1990.

Data derived from small sampling intervals should be interpreted with caution, and one should resist the tendency to use breath-by-breath data simply because the technology is available. Breath-by-breath sampling can be invaluable for certain research applications, such as when measuring oxygen kinetics or when end-tidal pressures are needed, but it is inappropriate for general clinical applications. Breath averaging would appear to represent a reasonable balance between precision (when high precision is needed) and variability. For most clinical uses, the variability associated with samples less than 30 sec is unacceptably high. We find it useful to configure the system to report the test results using 30-sec samples printed every 10 sec. This smooths the data, yet permits adequate resolution for choosing test endpoints, the ventilatory threshold, and other relevant analysis points. Regardless of the sample chosen, investigators should report the sampling interval used, and the intervals should be consistent throughout a given trial when one is studying an intervention.

NONINVASIVE DETERMINATION OF CARDIAC OUTPUT

With invasive exercise testing (chapter 7) the accurate measurement of cardiac output is easy; mixed venous oxygen concentration can be obtained from a catheter in the pulmonary artery, arterial oxygen content can be obtained from a catheter in the radial artery, and oxygen uptake can be measured with a metabolic system placed in the catheterization laboratory. Cardiac output determined directly by this method is the standard against which the other methods are compared. However, for obvious reasons this is usually reserved for patients who are undergoing catheterization for clinical purposes. Noninvasive methods have been developed to estimate cardiac output using gas exchange techniques. Two widely used techniques are based on the application of $\dot{V}CO_2$, rather than $\dot{V}O_2$, to the Fick equation:

$$\text{Cardiac output} = \frac{\dot{V}CO_2}{\text{a-v}CO_2 \text{ difference}},$$

where $\dot{V}CO_2$ is the volume of carbon dioxide produced, and a-vCO_2 difference is the difference in the CO_2 content between the arterial and venous blood.

$\dot{V}CO_2$ is easily measured during exercise with a metabolic system. To obtain cardiac output, the challenge concerns accurate measurements of arterial and venous CO_2 content. The easiest way to obtain arterial CO_2 content is to draw an arterial blood gas sample. Arterial CO_2 content (in ml/100 ml or percent) can be derived from the PCO_2 of the arterial blood sample using a standard CO_2 dissociation curve (Figure 3.8). Naturally, arterial blood gases are invasive, costly, and inconvenient, and they are not indicated for most subjects. An alternative is to

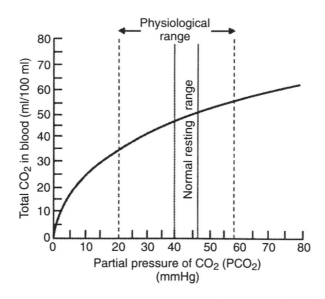

Figure 3.8   The CO_2 dissociation curve with the normal operating range. The CO_2 carried in the blood depends primarily on the partial pressure of CO_2. The relationship is nearly linear within the physiological range. Arterial CO_2 content is derived from the PCO_2 of the blood using either a blood gas sample or a CO_2 rebreathing technique.

estimate arterial PCO_2 noninvasively from the end-tidal PCO_2 using the following equation (2):

$$P_aCO_2 = 5.5 + 0.90(P_{ET}CO_2) - 0.0021(V_T),$$

where $P_{ET}CO_2$ is the end-tidal PCO_2 and V_T is the tidal volume.

Similarly, venous CO_2 content can be obtained noninvasively by using the lung as a surrogate for the blood. This requires rebreathing a gas mixture from a bag with a higher than normal CO_2 content, until either the gas in the bag and alveolar gas are in equilibrium (and therefore equal to venous blood) or the rate of rise in the CO_2 content in the lung during rebreathing can be extrapolated to equal that of the venous blood. Both these techniques are outlined below.

There are several advantages to these methods of measuring cardiac output. First, it can be done noninvasively (some laboratories add a single blood gas sample, i.e., for pH, hemoglobin, oxygen saturation, or P_aCO_2, but these can be assumed for most individuals exercising in a submaximal **steady state**). Second, although some of the particulars have been disputed, studies are available on the validity and reproducibility of the technique (3-10). Third, it is simple to perform and therefore can be repeated several times during a single steady-state bout of work. Fourth, all three variables needed to derive cardiac output by the Fick principle can be determined with a single metabolic system, a system which is no different from that used for a standard gas exchange test. Specialized software for this procedure may be helpful, and many of the commercially available systems provide this option. A disadvantage of this technology is that it is only valid during a steady metabolic state, making it unusable at higher levels of exercise.

The two commonly used methods that employ rebreathing techniques to determine cardiac output are an "equilibrium" method described by Collier in 1956 (11) and an "exponential" method described by Defares in 1958 (12).

Equilibrium Method

This method employs a rebreathing bag with a gas mixture containing a high concentration of CO_2 (9% to 14%). Normally, blood returned to the pulmonary circulation from the working muscles has a high CO_2 content (i.e., PCO_2 of the venous blood equals approximately 46 mmHg). As air enters the lung, a concentration gradient dictates that CO_2 leaves the venous blood (PCO_2 of the alveolar capillaries equals approximately 40 mmHg), enters the pulmonary circulation, and is exhaled. When the subject begins rebreathing from a bag with a high CO_2 content, it causes the lung to contain as much or more CO_2 as the venous blood, which results in a reversal of the normal concentration gradient. After a series of breaths (10 to 15 sec), the CO_2 gradient that has been reversed will come into equilibrium with the blood passing through the lungs. At this point, alveolar PCO_2 will equal that of the mixed venous blood entering the lung (and that moving in and out of the mouth from the bag). The assumption is made that no net transfer occurs across the pulmonary membrane. The equilibrium between alveolar air and mixed venous blood is indicated by a plateau in the recording of CO_2 concentration (Figure 3.9). It is this CO_2 tension that is used as an estimate of PCO_2 in the venous blood, completing the Fick equation.

Exponential Method

This method employs the same principle as the equilibrium technique; i.e., CO_2 is applied to the Fick equation. The rebreathing gas mixture contains a lower concentration of CO_2, often on the order of 4%, with an O_2 concentration of roughly 35%, and the balance nitrogen. Using this gas concentration, the blood leaving the lung has a high CO_2 content, and as the blood passes through the tissues, additional CO_2 is added. As the blood recirculates, venous CO_2 increases. The PCO_2 of the venous blood is estimated by plotting the rise in end-tidal carbon dioxide pressure with each breath and extrapolating a line to a point representing an equilibrium between the CO_2 pressure in the alveolar air and the blood (Figure 3.10). Complete recirculation occurs in approximately 10 to 15 sec. In a refinement of this method outlined by da Silva et al. (13), a computer-derived best fit curve for the exponential rise in CO_2 was most precise when solved for 20 sec.

Although used on a limited basis in the clinical setting, these noninvasive methods for determining cardiac output have great potential for use in a variety of settings including clinical and research applications. Generally, the only additional equipment needed involves the proper gas mixture, a rebreathing bag, and the proper valve apparatus to switch quickly from room air to the rebreathing bag. Detailed reviews are available in terms of the technique's history, methodology, validity, and reliability (3,4).

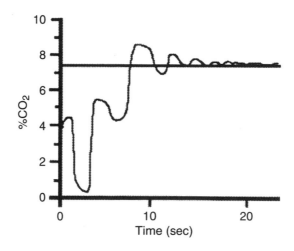

Figure 3.9   Equilibrium curve obtained during steady-state exercise for the CO_2 rebreathing technique described in Collier (11).

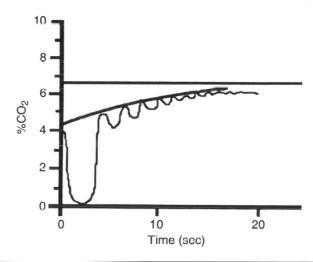

Figure 3.10 Exponential curve obtained during steady-state exercise for the CO_2 rebreathing method described in Defares (12).

DATA VALIDATION AND QUALITY CONTROL

Gas exchange analysis is an imperfect science. Considerable errors can occur if specific procedures are not followed to minimize them. To ensure that the data obtained are valid, the technician must possess some basic skills in gas exchange analysis, maintain quality control, and have the ability to identify errors and the reasons underlying them. With a little experience, errors and their sources can be identified quickly and rectified. It is important to be able to identify errors in the calibration before the test, as well as errors that may occur during the test and while interpreting the results. The reliability and accuracy of an analyzer are only as good as the calibration techniques employed. Moreover, the calibration procedure is meaningless if the calibration gas is unreliable. We have seen a number of recent multicenter pharmaceutical trials in cardiovascular disease attempt to incorporate gas exchange data in the study results but fail miserably because the data were unacceptable due to inconsistencies in calibration, lack of technical experience, and the absence of quality control at the different hospitals. Studies have documented inconsistencies in gas exchange data among laboratories in both Britain and Canada (14,15). These studies have suggested that variations between laboratories as high as 25% can occur, which probably are attributable to a lack of attention paid to quality control.

Gas analyzers and flow meters are prone to drift. This can occur from day to day and even from test to test. It is therefore essential that the system be calibrated immediately before each test is performed. Following the test, the analyzers should be checked again to identify any errors that may have caused the data to be invalid. Because ambient conditions can affect the concentration of oxygen in the inspired air, it is necessary to have a thermometer, barometer, and hygrometer in the laboratory. A fan is useful when the laboratory is small or when flow is measured with a pneumotach or turbine system at the mouth. This ensures a reasonable fraction of inspired oxygen. A record of the calibration results should accompany each test; valid interpretation of test results is possible only in the presence of appropriate calibration values. Modern gas exchange systems that are commercially available have convenient calibration procedures controlled by a microprocessor. The calibration procedure should include documentation of the ambient environment and the accuracy of airflow and both the oxygen and carbon dioxide analyzers (Table 3.1).

Metabolic systems are a little like your car: most of its parts have a finite lifetime, and it occasionally needs a tuneup. For example, with frequent use, a zirconium electrochemical cell oxygen analyzer can only be expected to last

Table 3.1   Information That Calibration Report Should Contain

---

AMBIENT ENVIRONMENT
- Temperature
- Barometric pressure
- Relative humidity
- O_2 concentration (%)
- CO_2 concentration (%)

EQUIPMENT SPECIFICATIONS
- O_2 concentration in calibration tank
- CO_2 concentration in calibration tank
- Valve dead space
- Syringe size for volume calibration

SYSTEM PERFORMANCE
- Volume:
  Flow meter measured volume
  Calibration factor
  Deviation (% error)
- O_2 analyzer:
  % O_2 measured from calibration gas
  Deviation (% error)
  System response time or "phase delay"
  Ambient O_2 during calibration test or response test
- CO_2 analyzer:
  % CO_2 measured from calibration gas
  Deviation (% error)
  System response time or "phase delay"
  Ambient CO_2 during calibration test or response test

ROUTINES TO KNOW:
GENERAL CALIBRATION PROCEDURES

As systems differ, the specific calibration protocol outlined by the manufacturer should be carefully followed. A recent American Heart Association Task Force statement on setting up an exercise laboratory (16) lists the following general calibration procedures in order to ensure that valid data are obtained:

1. The exercise laboratory should be well ventilated; a fan is helpful. Room air should read $20.93 \pm 0.03\%$ O_2 at 0% humidity. However, the precise fraction is dependent upon ambient conditions and should be adjusted accordingly. A calibration source containing 100% N_2 should read 0% O_2. The analyzer should be checked further by simulating the fraction of expired O_2 (F_EO_2) during the test, i.e., approximately 16% O_2. Since this is essentially a validation of system linearity, the concentration of O_2 in the calibration tank is not important as long as it is in the range of the expected exhaled air. However, it is essential that the actual concentration in the tank is known precisely, and this should be verified by the distributor or, if possible, checked independently with a mass spectrometer.

2. The CO_2 analyzer should read a room air fraction of $0.03 \pm 0.2\%$ (essentially zero) and should not change when the 100% N_2 or simulated F_EO_2 fractions are sampled from the calibration tanks. The CO_2 analyzer should likewise be checked further by simulating the fraction of expired CO_2 (F_ECO_2) during exercise, i.e., approximately 4% CO_2.

3. For breath-by-breath systems, it is also preferable to check the O_2 and CO_2 analyzer response times or "delays." It is important that the system meets the specifications outlined by the manufacturer. Most manufacturers make this feature available.

4. Once limited to large weather balloons and Tissots, great strides have been made in the measurement of ventilatory volume, and numerous flow devices are now available, including small turbines, propellers, and even disposable pneumotachs. All can be validated before testing by ascertaining a stable baseline (0 L/min) and injecting a known volume (usually 3 or 4 L from a syringe). It is preferable to perform several injections at different flow rates to ensure stability. The average error should be within $\pm 3\%$ of the known volume.

about 1.5 years, and ancillary parts are certain to give out in the meantime. Therefore, when purchasing a metabolic system, the company's ability to provide technical service should be a strong consideration. Even the most experienced user will at times find it necessary to contact the manufacturer's service department for assistance with technical problems. Whenever possible, a service contract should be included when negotiating the purchase of a system. A good service contract should include immediate technical support by telephone, a warranty on parts, and local technical support if necessary.

System Validation

In addition to pretest calibration procedures, other methods can be employed to validate the system on a routine basis. Gas exchange variables are highly reproducible within a given subject. We have effectively used a protocol recommended by Jones (17) in which laboratory staff members are tested at submaximal steady-state workloads periodically. It is recommended that several staff members participate in this process, each using a somewhat different steady-state workload, and that these procedures be performed monthly. Oxygen uptake, ventilation, and CO_2 production should be reproducible from test to test for a given subject within ± 5%. Besides being reproducible, the data should approximate the predicted oxygen cost of a given steady-state workload (± 10%). (See appendix A for estimating the oxygen cost of work.)

A clever calibration device that has recently become available is a gas exchange validator developed by Huszczuk et al. (18) and distributed by the Medical Graphics Corporation (St. Paul, MN). This system simulates a wide range of respiratory gas exchange rates for on-line calibration of metabolic systems. It employs a pump that takes in a mixture of room air and a known volume of calibration gas. It then expels a gas mixture at a concentration and volume that resemble those of normal human respiration. The mixture of ''inspired'' air and flow rate can be set to simulate any given metabolic rate. This system is easy to use and is accurate within ± 2%. Routine use of such a system would greatly facilitate the calibration process, and it would increase confidence in gas exchange responses considerably. While its use is limited now, it seems imminent that this or devices similar to it will become the norm for validation and calibration of metabolic systems.

Other Sources of Error

Aside from the flow meter or gas analyzers, other common sources of error include a leaking valve, mouthpiece, or face mask or a blockage in the sample line caused by a kink or dust accumulation. Many sources of error can be identified while collecting resting data from the patient before the test. A resting period of 1 to 5 min not only identifies most errors before starting but also provides the opportunity to ascertain that the test begins with the patient in a relaxed, basal state. Inappropriate gas exchange responses may also be observed when the treadmill or cycle ergometer is not calibrated properly. Procedures for treadmill and cycle ergometer calibration follow.

ROUTINES TO KNOW: CALIBRATION OF TREADMILL SPEED AND ELEVATION

Treadmill Speed. Calibration of treadmill speed requires knowledge of the belt length, which can be obtained from the manufacturer or measured with a tape. The treadmill speed can be calibrated by counting the number of rotations of the treadmill belt per unit of time. Using a mark on the treadmill belt as a reference, the number of belt revolutions in 1 min can be counted, and knowing the length of the belt, the actual miles per hour can be calculated by

$$\frac{\text{Belt length (inches)} \times \text{number of revolutions/min}}{1056},$$

where 1056 is the conversion of inches per minute to miles per hour.

The value obtained is the treadmill speed in miles per hour. If the speed indicator does not agree with this value, adjust the meter to the proper setting. Frequently a calibration adjustment screw is accessible through a small opening in the front of the control panel. If this option is not available, contact the manufacturer. The calibration procedure should be repeated at several speeds to ascertain accuracy across commonly employed protocols in a given laboratory.

Treadmill Elevation. Calibration of treadmill elevation is performed by measuring a fixed distance on the floor and determining the difference in height of the treadmill over the fixed distance. The following specific procedures are performed:

1. Using a carpenter's level, make certain that the treadmill is resting on a level surface. If the surface is not level, shims may be placed under the treadmill supports to achieve the proper "zero" reference with the carpenter's level. Set the treadmill elevation to 0% grade. If the elevation does not read 0% when it is level, adjust the potentiometer until it does.

2. Mark two points 20 inches apart along the length of the treadmill.

3. Elevate the treadmill to its metered reading of 20% grade and measure the distance of each of the two points to the floor.

4. Divide the difference between the two heights by 20. The results should be .20, or 20%, when the elevation is properly calibrated. If the result is not 20%, adjust the elevation meter potentiometer so that it reads the elevation percentage that was calculated. A check of 5, 10, and 15% grade readings is recommended to ensure the validity of intermediate positions.

(continued)

ROUTINES TO KNOW *(continued)*

Calibrate speed and elevation without a subject on the treadmill. Following calibration, however, ask a moderately heavy subject of 75 to 100 kg (165 to 220 pounds) to walk on the treadmill to ensure that the calibrations remain accurate when in use. Speed should remain unchanged regardless of the weight of the individual on the treadmill.

After approximately 1,000 hours of use, the treadmill should be fully serviced. Lubricate motor bearings, check the variable speed belt for wear, center the belt, grease the chain drive, and clean and lubricate the gears. Service and maintenance schedules should be available from the manufacturer.

Treadmill and Cycle Ergometer Calibration

When the exercise testing equipment is out of calibration, not only is the workload administered unknown but the validation procedures among staff members outlined above are useless. Specific directions for calibration and preventive maintenance are frequently available in the manufacturer's operations manual. It is a good practice to perform calibration procedures monthly and to keep a record of the dates they were performed along with the results.

Bicycle Ergometer Calibration

Since the work rate on a mechanically braked ergometer depends not only on the resistance but also on the cycling rate in revolutions per minute, a counter is needed to quantify RPMs. It is also important to adjust belt tension appropriately and to clean the flywheel to ensure smooth operation. Electrically braked ergometers are more difficult to calibrate and require special instruments generally not available to the individual purchaser, so calibration is usually provided by the manufacturer or by the institutional biomedical engineering department.

SUMMARY

A basic understanding of theory, calculations, and instrumentation is critical to cardiopulmonary exercise testing. Acquiring oxygen uptake during exercise requires knowledge of three variables: the fraction of oxygen in the inspired air, the fraction of oxygen in the expired air, and the volume of the inspired or expired air. Carbon dioxide must also be analyzed in order to correct for differences in

ROUTINES TO KNOW:
CALIBRATION OF CYCLE ERGOMETERS

Mechanically Braked Cycle Ergometers. To check the calibration on a mechanically braked cycle ergometer (such as a Monarch or Tunturi), perform the following routine:

1. Remove the belt from the wheel.

2. Set the mark on the pendulum weight at zero and attach an accurate weight to the belt. The weight should hang freely. A reading of that weight should be given accurately on the scale.

3. If all conditions are met and the scale continues to show an incorrect reading for the known weight, turn the adjusting screw until the scale reads the appropriate weight.

Lateral Friction Braked Ergometers. When calibrating an ergometer that is braked by a lateral friction device, use the following routine:

1. Place the ergometer on two chairs so that the brake scale plate is vertical.

2. After releasing the brake regulator knob on the handlebar, hang a known metric weight on the brake arm using a wire S-hook to attach the weight.

3. Loosen the fastening screw of the shock absorber at one end. The scale should now read, in kiloponds, the exact amount of the weight attached to the brake arm. Always read the pointer directly from above.

4. If the scale does not accurately read the weight, turn the regulating nut. When the pointer indicates the same figure as the weight attached, the ergometer is correctly calibrated.

Mechanically braked ergometers can be delicate and may lose adjustment during frequent use or if transported. Before using an ergometer, check the chain for tightness and lubrication and clean the braking surfaces. To smooth the braking surface, press a fine sandpaper against it while pedaling the ergometer.

the inspired and expired volumes. The collection of expired ventilation has been greatly simplified in recent years and is commonly measured using a *pneumotachometer*. As a rule, gas exchange variables pertaining to volumes within the lungs are expressed body temperature and pressure, saturated (BTPS), and those involving the exchange of gas in the bloodstream are expressed standard temperature and pressure, dry (STPD).

The basic elements of noninvasive gas exchange techniques can be used to determine cardiac output by application of carbon dioxide to the Fick equation. The challenge in doing so involves obtaining an estimate of venous CO_2 content. This requires rebreathing a CO_2 mixture from a bag until the gas in the bag is in equilibrium with the alveolar gas (or an extrapolation for such is made). The introduction of microprocessors into the exercise laboratory has greatly facilitated the acquisition of these and other cardiopulmonary measurements.

Strict attention to quality control is essential to ensure that valid data are obtained. Common sources of error in cardiopulmonary exercise testing include an oxygen or carbon dioxide analyzer that is out of calibration, a flow meter with an unstable baseline, a treadmill or cycle ergometer that is out of calibration, or a leaking valve, face mask, or mouthpiece. Performing system analyzer calibration procedures outlined by the manufacturer before every test can alleviate most problems encountered when using a metabolic system.

REFERENCES

1. Myers J, Walsh D, Sullivan M, Froelicher VF. 1990. Effect of sampling on variability and plateau in oxygen uptake. J Appl Physiol 68: 404-410.
2. McEvoy JE, Jones NL. 1975. Arterialized capillary blood gases in exercise studies. Med Sci Sports 7: 312-315.
3. Kirby TE. 1985. The CO_2 rebreathing technique for determination of cardiac output: Part 1. J Cardiac Rehabil 5: 97-101.
4. Kirby TE. 1985. The CO_2 rebreathing technique for determination of cardiac output: Part 2. J Cardiac Rehabil 5: 132-138.
5. Heigenhauser GF, Jones NL. 1979. Comparison of two rebreathing methods for the determination of mixed venous partial pressure carbon dioxide during exercise. Clin Sci 56: 433-437.
6. Forster RE. 1977. Can alveolar PCO_2 exceed pulmonary end-capillary CO_2? No. J Appl Physiol 42: 323-328.
7. Gurtner GH. 1977. Can alveolar PCO_2 exceed pulmonary end-capillary CO_2? Yes. J Appl Physiol 42: 324-326.
8. Franciosa JA, Ragan DO, Rubenstone SJ. 1976. Validation of the CO_2 rebreathing method for measuring cardiac output in patients with hypertension or heart failure. J Lab Clin Med 88: 627.
9. Franciosa JA. 1977. Evaluation of the CO_2 rebreathing cardiac output method in seriously ill patients. Circulation 55: 449.
10. Ferguson RJ, Faulkner JA, Julius S, Conway J. 1968. Comparison of cardiac output determined by CO_2 rebreathing and dye-dilution methods. J Appl Physiol 25: 450.

11. Collier CR. 1956. Determination of mixed venous CO_2 tensions by rebreathing. J Appl Physiol 9: 25-29.
12. Defares JG. 1958. Determination of $PVCO_2$ from the exponential CO_2 use during rebreathing. J Appl Physiol 13: 159-164.
13. da Silva GA, El-Manshawi A, Heigenhauser GJF, Jones NL. 1985. Measurement of mixed venous carbon dioxide pressure by rebreathing during exercise. J Appl Physiol 59: 379-392.
14. Contes JE, Woolmer RE. 1962. A comparison between 27 laboratories of the results of analysis of an expired gas sample. J Physiol 163: 36P-37P.
15. Jones NL, Kane JW. 1979. Quality control of exercise test measurements. Med Sci Sports 11: 368-372.
16. Pina IL, Balady GJ, Hanson P, Labovitz AJ, Madonna DW, Myers J. 1995. Guidelines for clinical exercise testing laboratories. A statement from the American Heart Association Committee on Exercise and Cardiac Rehabilitation. Circulation 91: 912-921.
17. Jones NL. 1988. Clinical Exercise Testing, 210. Philadelphia: Saunders.
18. Huszczuk A, Whipp BJ, Wasserman K. 1990. A respiratory gas exchange simulator for routine calibration in metabolic studies. Eur Resp J 3: 465-468.

INFORMATION FROM VENTILATORY GAS EXCHANGE DATA

*M*aximal oxygen uptake is the most common and most important measurement derived from gas exchange data during exercise. Unfortunately, it is frequently the only variable used in many laboratories. Gas exchange techniques can provide a great deal of additional information regarding the capacity of the heart and lungs to deliver oxygen to the working muscle during exercise. In this chapter, maximal oxygen uptake and other gas exchange variables are outlined with particular emphasis on their applications to testing patients with heart disease. For reference, formulas for calculating these variables are outlined in Table 4.1.

The benefits of adding gas exchange techniques to the standard exercise test have been emphasized repeatedly thus far. It is worth mentioning again that there is no more accurate or reproducible measure of cardiopulmonary function

Table 4.1 Calculations for Basic Gas Exchange Data

1. Oxygen uptake ($\dot{V}O_2$, L/min, STPD) $= \left[\dfrac{(1 - F_EO_2 - F_ECO_2)}{.7904} \times (F_IO_2 - F_EO_2) \right]$
$\times \dot{V}_E$ (STPD)

2. Minute ventilation ($\dot{V}_E$, L/min, BTPS) = respiratory rate × tidal volume. For calculations of $\dot{V}O_2$ and $\dot{V}CO_2$, $\dot{V}_E$ in BTPS is converted to STPD by the following:
$$\dot{V}_E \text{ (L/min, STPD)} = \dot{V}_E \text{ (L/min, BTPS)} \times \frac{273}{(273 + 37)} \times \frac{(Pb - 47)}{760}$$
or $\dot{V}_E$ (L/min, STPD) $= \dot{V}_E$ (L/min, BTPS) × 0.826 if Pb = 760 mmHg

3. Carbon dioxide production ($\dot{V}CO_2$, L/min, STPD) $= \dot{V}_E$ (L/min, STPD) × F_ECO_2

4. Respiratory exchange ratio (RER) $= \dfrac{\dot{V}CO_2 \text{ (L/min, STPD)}}{\dot{V}O_2 \text{ (L/min, STPD)}}$

5. Oxygen pulse (O_2 pulse, ml O_2/beat) $= \dfrac{\dot{V}O_2 \text{ (ml/min, STPD)}}{\text{heart rate (beats/min)}}$

6. Ventilatory equivalents for O_2 and CO_2 $= \dfrac{\dot{V}_E \text{ (L/min, BTPS)}}{\dot{V}O_2 \text{ (L/min, STPD)}}$ and
$\dfrac{\dot{V}_E \text{ (L/min, BTPS)}}{\dot{V}CO_2 \text{ (L/min, STPD)}}$

7. End-tidal PCO_2 ($P_{ET}CO_2$, mmHg) $= F_{ET}CO_2 \times (Pb - 47)$

8. Ventilatory dead space (V_D, L) $= V_T$ (L) $\times \dfrac{(P_aCO_2 - P_ECO_2)}{P_aCO_2}$
$-$ valve dead space (L)
where $P_ECO_2 = F_ECO_2 \times (Pb - 47)$ and P_aCO_2 is estimated using
$P_aCO_2 = 5.5 + 0.90 \ P_{ET}CO_2 - .0021 \ V_T$
The ventilatory dead space to tidal volume ratio (V_D/V_T) is calculated by dividing by V_T.

9. Aveolar-arterial PO_2 difference $= [P(A-a)O_2]$
P_aO_2 obtained from arterial blood gas
P_AO_2 (room air) $= [(Pb - 47) \times 0.2093] - \dfrac{P_aCO_2}{RER}$

10. Breathing reserve $= \dfrac{\text{Maximal } \dot{V}_E \text{ (L/min)}}{\text{MVV (L/min)}}$
where $\dot{V}E$ is calculated using equation 2 and MVV is the maximal voluntary ventilation at rest.

BTPS = body temperature and pressure, saturated. Gas volume at body temperature and pressure saturated with water vapor (37 °C and 47 mmHg). STPD = standard temperature and pressure, dry. Gas volume at standard temperature (0 °C) and barometric pressure (760 mmHg), dry. Pb = barometric pressure, mmHg. V_T = tidal volume, ml. $P_{ET}O_2$ = end-tidal oxygen pressure, mmHg. $P_{ET}CO_2$ = end-tidal carbon dioxide pressure, mmHg. P_ECO_2 = mixed expired carbon dioxide pressure, mmHg. P_aCO_2 = partial pressure of carbon dioxide in arterial blood. F_EO_2 = fraction (%) of oxygen in the expired air. F_ECO_2 = fraction (%) of carbon dioxide in the expired air. F_IO_2 = fraction (%) of oxygen in the inspired air. F_ICO_2 = fraction (%) of carbon dioxide in the inspired air. P_aO_2 = partial pressure of arterial oxygen. P_AO_2 = partial pressure of alveolar oxygen.

than directly measured oxygen uptake. With a little experience using the technology, one gains a sense of what is normally observed both submaximally and maximally in a given condition. Abnormalities in ventilatory gas exchange in certain conditions can be invaluable when evaluating interventions. However, like all medical tests, exercise testing is an imperfect procedure. Even combinations of ancillary exercise techniques (echo, nuclear, and pharmacologic stress [1-3]) can be misleading a certain percentage of the time. The gas exchange exercise test is no exception. Regardless of any apparent abnormality or what might be expected for a given patient, there is significant overlap between what constitutes normal or abnormal. The examples that come to mind immediately are the coronary disease patients who are asymptomatic and achieve a high level of fitness (4) or the patients with chronic heart failure who, despite poor ventricular function, demonstrate a normal $\dot{V}O_2$max and none of the other gas exchange abnormalities that are typical of heart failure patients (5). On the other end of the spectrum and contrary to common perception, maximal oxygen uptake is only a modest predictor of endurance performance among athletes; this measurement varies considerably among individuals whose performance is similar at the elite level (6,7). When using gas exchange techniques, we have therefore found it generally preferable to avoid dichotomous cut points for abnormal, the use of algorithms, and "magic numbers" often used by practitioners who are well versed in this area.

MAXIMAL OXYGEN UPTAKE

$\dot{V}O_2$max is an objective measurement of exercise capacity: it defines the upper limits of the cardiopulmonary system. It is determined by the capacity to increase heart rate, augment stroke volume, and direct blood flow to the active muscles. It is often the most important variable measured, although this depends on the setting and the context of the particular patient being tested. $\dot{V}O_2$max should initially be considered in terms of what is normal for a given individual if he or she were healthy. Determining what constitutes "normal" is no small task (this is covered in more detail in chapter 6). Generally, however, the observation that $\dot{V}O_2$max falls within the normal range for a given gender and age makes a strong and multifactorial statement, i.e., that the individual has no significant impairment in the cardiopulmonary system. Implicit with this statement, of course, is that the patient has no major limitations to cardiac output, its redistribution, or skeletal muscle metabolism or function. Changes in $\dot{V}O_2$max following training or detraining or those caused by disease closely parallel changes in cardiac size and maximal cardiac output (8-10). Clearly, $\dot{V}O_2$max is directly related to the integrated function of several systems.

Although the process has been slow, a better appreciation for directly measured $\dot{V}O_2$max is evolving in clinical cardiology. For example, a number of pharmaceutical companies, recognizing the limitations in exercise time as a measure of cardiopulmonary work (see chapter 1), have recently employed gas exchange techniques in large multicenter trials (11). The clinical importance of an objective and accurate measurement of exercise capacity is underscored by studies on prognosis in patients with heart disease. Exercise capacity has consistently been an important predictor of prognosis. In a recent review, exercise capacity was chosen more frequently than any other variable (including the patient's clinical history, markers of ischemia, or other exercise test variables) as a significant determinant of survival (12).

Mancini and co-workers (13) recently studied 114 candidates for cardiac transplantation and found that peak $\dot{V}O_2$ was the best predictor of survival, with only pulmonary capillary wedge pressure providing additional prognostic information. Patients awaiting transplantation who achieved a peak $\dot{V}O_2 \geq$ 14 ml/kg/min had a 1-year survival rate of 94%, whereas among those achieving < 14 ml/kg/min, the survival rate was only 47%. Needless to say, the more imprecise measure of work, treadmill time, could not have separated patients so clearly. This is one example in which an important clinical decision (who should receive a transplant and when) was facilitated by gas exchange techniques. Vanhees et al. (14) recently studied 527 patients referred for cardiac rehabilitation over a 10-year period and observed that peak oxygen uptake had a strong inverse association with cardiovascular death. Other generally accepted indicators of risk such as blood lipids, family history of heart disease, blood pressure, chest pain during exercise, and ventricular arrhythmias did not predict mortality. Nixon et al. (15) compared the prognostic value of clinical markers of disease severity in patients with cystic fibrosis with peak oxygen uptake: they found the latter to be the most important predictor of mortality. While higher peak oxygen uptake is no doubt a marker for less severe illness, these studies nevertheless suggest an important role for measured oxygen uptake in determining prognosis.

MINUTE VENTILATION

Minute ventilation ($\dot{V}_E$) is the volume of air moving into and out of the lungs expressed in liters per minute (BTPS). It is determined by the product of respiratory rate and the volume of air exhaled with each breath (the tidal volume). The product of ventilation and true O_2 (the difference between inspired and expired oxygen content) determines oxygen uptake. Because true O_2 generally changes by similar amounts among normal individuals, ventilation is the major component of oxygen uptake during exercise. Fit individuals with high maximal ventilations and thus high values for maximal oxygen uptake, however, must also have high maximal cardiac outputs that match ventilation in the lungs. The ratio of alveolar ventilation to alveolar capillary blood flow, termed the **ventilation-perfusion ratio**, is roughly 0.80 at rest. With exercise, ventilation and alveolar blood flow increase such that this ratio may approach 5.0. Abnormal ventilation is an important characteristic of patients with chronic heart failure and pulmonary disease, due in part to a mismatching of ventilation and perfusion. The ventilatory response to exercise in patients with chronic heart failure has been of particular interest in recent years, and gas exchange data can be important in identifying the degree of impairment in these patients and in gauging their response to therapy.

Pulmonary ventilation is equal to the sum of the air that participates in gas exchange (alveolar ventilation, V_A) and air that does not, i.e., the dead space (V_D). The dead space reflects air in the conducting airways and nonperfused alveoli:

$$V_E = V_A + V_D$$

The dead space fraction of ventilation is commonly expressed relative to tidal volume (V_D/V_T). The V_D/V_T determines the difference between V_E and V_A:

$$V_A - V_E \times (1 - V_D/V_T)$$

Because ventilation has the primary responsibility of clearing CO_2 from the blood, the volume of ventilation is also determined by carbon dioxide production ($\dot{V}CO_2$) and arterial CO_2 pressure (P_aCO_2). The three factors that dictate the quantity of ventilation can be expressed by the following:

$$\dot{V}_E = \frac{863\ \dot{V}CO_2}{P_aCO_2 \times (1 - V_D/V_T)}$$

where 863 is a constant necessary to convert $\dot{V}_E$ to BTPS conditions ($\dot{V}_E$ is expressed in L/min, BTPS, and $\dot{V}CO_2$ is expressed in L/min, STPD).

CARBON DIOXIDE PRODUCTION

Carbon dioxide produced by the body ($\dot{V}CO_2$) during exercise is expressed in liters per minute, STPD. $\dot{V}CO_2$ is generated from two sources during exercise. One source, the metabolic CO_2, is produced by oxidative metabolism. Roughly 75% of the oxygen consumed by the body is converted to carbon dioxide, which is returned to the right heart by the venous blood, enters the lungs, and is exhaled as $\dot{V}CO_2$. A second source of CO_2 is often called nonmetabolic and results from the buffering of lactate at higher levels of exercise. An elevation in carbon dioxide in the blood can quickly result in respiratory acidosis. Fortunately, the major determinants of ventilation during exercise are these two sources of CO_2 in the blood, which are reflected in the expired air as $\dot{V}CO_2$. Thus, $\dot{V}CO_2$ closely matches $\dot{V}_E$ during exercise, and the body maintains a relatively normal pH under most conditions. $\dot{V}CO_2$ and $\dot{V}_E$ also parallel increases in $\dot{V}O_2$ or work rate during exercise levels up to roughly 50% to 70% of $\dot{V}O_2$max. At exercise levels beyond this, $\dot{V}_E$ increases disproportionately to $\dot{V}O_2$. This is because as exercise increases in intensity, lactate is produced at a greater rate than it is removed from the blood. The lactate must be buffered, and this process yields an additional source CO_2, which stimulates ventilation. This "ventilatory threshold" has generated a great deal of interest over the years.

The fraction of expired carbon dioxide ($F_E CO_2$) is, of course, a function of the total ventilation and carbon dioxide production:

$$F_E CO_2\ (\%) = \frac{\dot{V}CO_2}{\dot{V}_E}$$

When expressing expired carbon dioxide as a partial pressure, the equation becomes

$$P_E CO_2\ (mmHg) = \frac{\dot{V}CO_2 \times 863}{\dot{V}_E}$$

where 863 is a correction for $\dot{V}_E$ under BTPS conditions ($\dot{V}CO_2$ is in L/min, STPD, and $\dot{V}_E$ is in L/min, BTPS).

RESPIRATORY EXCHANGE RATIO

The respiratory exchange ratio (RER) represents the amount of carbon dioxide produced divided by the amount of oxygen consumed. Roughly 75% of the oxygen consumed is converted to carbon dioxide. Thus, RER at rest generally ranges from 0.75 to 0.85. Because RER depends on the type of fuel used by the cells, it can provide an index of carbohydrate or fat metabolism. If carbohydrates were the predominant fuel, RER would equal 1.0 given the formula:

$$C_6H_{12}O_6\ (glucose) + 6O_2 \rightleftarrows 6CO_2 + 6H_2O$$

$$RER = \dot{V}CO_2\ divided\ by\ \dot{V}O_2 = 6CO_2\ divided\ by\ 6O_2 = 1.0$$

Because more oxygen is required to burn fat, the respiratory exchange ratio for fat metabolism is lower, roughly 0.70. At high levels of exercise, CO_2 production exceeds oxygen uptake. Thus, an RER exceeding 1.0 to 1.2 is often used to indicate the subject is giving a maximal effort. However, peak RER values vary considerably and generally are not a precise cut point for "maximal" exercise.

It should be noted that in calculating the respiratory exchange ratio, the assumption is made that the exchange of O_2 and CO_2 measured in the lungs reflects the actual gas exchange from nutrient metabolism in the cell. This assumption is reasonably valid under most steady-state conditions, but several factors may disturb the normal relationship between these gases. For example, hyperventilation, by definition, is an increase in ventilation out of proportion to the metabolic demands, and greater expiration of CO_2 occurs, raising the respiratory exchange ratio. This rise in the respiratory exchange ratio cannot be attributed to greater carbohydrate oxidation.

OXYGEN PULSE

Oxygen pulse (O_2 pulse) is an indirect index of combined cardiopulmonary oxygen transport. It is calculated by dividing oxygen uptake (ml/min) by heart rate (beats/min). Normal values range from 4 to 6 at rest and generally increase to 10 to 20 with maximal effort. In effect, O_2 pulse is equal to the product of stroke volume and a-vO_2 difference. Thus, circulatory adjustments that occur during exercise (i.e., a widening of the a-vO_2 difference, increased cardiac output, and redistribution of blood flow to the working muscle) will increase O_2 pulse. Maximal O_2 pulse is higher in fitter subjects and lower in the presence of heart disease. More important, O_2 pulse is higher at any given workload in the fitter or healthier individual. Conversely, O_2 pulse will be reduced in any condition that reduces stroke volume (left ventricular dysfunction secondary to ischemia or infarction) or conditions that reduce arterial O_2 content (anemia, hypoxemia).

VENTILATORY EQUIVALENTS FOR OXYGEN AND CARBON DIOXIDE

The ventilatory equivalents for oxygen and carbon dioxide are calculated by dividing ventilation (L/min, BTPS) by $\dot{V}O_2$ and $\dot{V}CO_2$ (L/min, STPD), respectively. A large volume of ventilation (20 to 40 L) is required to consume a single liter of oxygen; thus, $\dot{V}_E/\dot{V}O_2$ is often in the 30s at rest. A decrease in $\dot{V}_E/\dot{V}O_2$ is normally observed from rest to a submaximal exercise level, followed by a rapid increase at higher levels of exercise when $\dot{V}_E$ increases in response to the need to buffer lactate (Figure 4.1). $\dot{V}_E/\dot{V}O_2$ reflects the ventilatory requirement for any given oxygen uptake; thus, it is an index of ventilatory efficiency. Patients with uneven matching of ventilation to perfusion in the lungs (a high fraction of physiologic dead space) ventilate inefficiently and have high values for $\dot{V}_E/\dot{V}O_2$. High $\dot{V}_E/\dot{V}O_2$ values characterize the response to exercise among patients with lung disease and/or chronic heart failure (Figure 4.2).

$\dot{V}_E/\dot{V}CO_2$ represents the ventilatory requirement to eliminate a given amount of CO_2 produced by the metabolizing tissues. Like the $\dot{V}_E/\dot{V}O_2$, it also reflects the dead space ventilation, but $\dot{V}_E/\dot{V}CO_2$ is strongly influenced by the P_aCO_2 as well. Since metabolic CO_2 is a strong stimulus for ventilation during exercise, $\dot{V}_E$ and $\dot{V}CO_2$ closely mirror one another, and after a drop in early exercise, $\dot{V}_E/\dot{V}CO_2$ normally does not increase significantly throughout submaximal exercise. However, in the presence of chronic heart failure, $\dot{V}_E/\dot{V}CO_2$ is shifted upward compared with that in normals, and high $\dot{V}_E/\dot{V}CO_2$ values are one characteristic of the abnormal ventilatory response to exercise in this condition. At low and moderate levels of exercise, the $\dot{V}_E/\dot{V}CO_2$ exceeds $\dot{V}_E/\dot{V}O_2$ as the respiratory exchange ratio is less than 1.0.

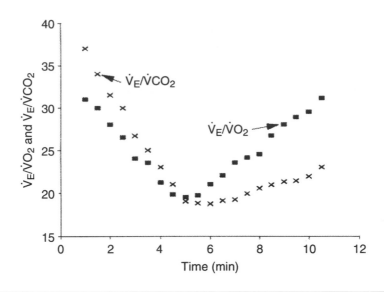

Figure 4.1 The response of the ventilatory equivalents for oxygen ($\dot{V}E/\dot{V}O_2$) and carbon dioxide ($\dot{V}_E/\dot{V}CO_2$) in a normal individual during a graded maximal exercise test.

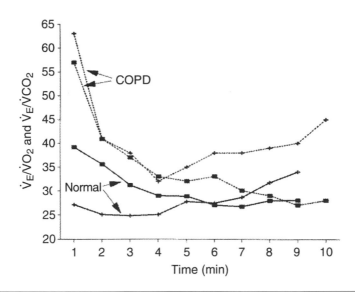

Figure 4.2 $\dot{V}_E/\dot{V}O_2$ (+) and $\dot{V}_E/\dot{V}CO_2$ (■) responses to exercise in two 44-year-old males, one with chronic obstructive pulmonary disease (COPD) and one normal. Both subjects performed maximal ramp protocols individualized to last approximately 10 min. Note the higher values for the patient and the breakpoints in ventilation relative to oxygen uptake in both subjects.

Caiozzo et al. (16) compared gas exchange indices used to detect the ventilatory threshold and found that the use of the ventilatory equivalents for O_2 and CO_2 most closely reflected a lactate inflection point and thus were the best indices to detect the ventilatory or lactate threshold. Many laboratories define the ventilatory threshold as the beginning of a systematic increase in $\dot{V}_E/\dot{V}O_2$ without an increase in $\dot{V}_E/\dot{V}CO_2$.

VENTILATORY DEAD SPACE TO TIDAL VOLUME RATIO

The ventilatory dead space to tidal volume ratio (V_D/V_T) ratio measured by gas exchange is an estimate of the fraction of tidal volume that represents physiologic dead space. Thus, it is another reflection of ventilatory efficiency. When estimating V_D/V_T, arterial carbon dioxide pressure is estimated from end-tidal carbon dioxide pressure. However, the end-tidal carbon dioxide pressure tends to overestimate arterial carbon dioxide pressure during exercise, resulting in V_D/V_T values that are erroneously high. On the other hand, when the dead space is elevated, the end-tidal carbon dioxide pressure will be lowered, leading to an underestimation of arterial carbon dioxide and subsequent underestimation of V_D/V_T. The estimation of arterial carbon dioxide pressure from gas exchange techniques can therefore be problematic in patients with airway or pulmonary vascular disease. Within these limitations, dead space estimated from gas exchange provides an indication of the contribution of dead space to $\dot{V}_E$. When an accurate measurement of V_D/V_T is important, however, arterial blood must be obtained directly to quantify arterial carbon dioxide pressure.

Physiologic dead space ventilation is the difference between minute ventilation and alveolar ventilation. Thus, V_D/V_T is an estimate of the degree to which ventilation matches perfusion in the lungs. V_D/V_T is low when there is a uniform matching of alveolar ventilation to perfusion. When significant ventilation-perfusion mismatching is present, V_D/V_T is high. In normal subjects, V_D/V_T falls from roughly one-third to between one-tenth and one-fifth at peak exercise. However, in the presence of pulmonary disease or heart failure, in which there can be significant ventilation-perfusion mismatching, V_D/V_T is elevated and can remain unchanged throughout exercise.

Ventilation-perfusion mismatching and thus a high V_D/V_T accounts in large part for the abnormally high ventilation observed in patients with pulmonary disease and heart failure. Figure 4.3 illustrates minute values for V_D/V_T throughout ramp exercise in a patient with chronic heart failure and a normal individual the same age. Although this particular patient achieved a relatively high peak $\dot{V}O_2$ value (19.0 ml/kg/min), more than half the tidal volume was attributable to physiologic dead space. With such a large fraction of dead space and thus

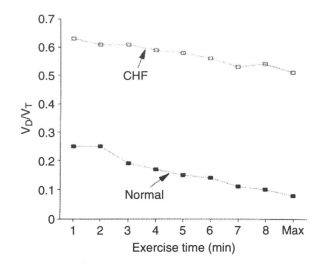

Figure 4.3   Minute values for V_D/V_T throughout ramp exercise in a patient with chronic heart failure (CHF) and a normal individual the same age. Ramp rates were individualized such that test duration was about 10 min for each subject. Note the considerably higher fraction of dead space in the patient. The patient achieved a relatively high peak $\dot{V}O_2$ of 19 ml/kg/min. However, with the high fraction of dead space, a great deal of ventilation was required to achieve this $\dot{V}O_2$, as evidenced by a high value for $\dot{V}_E/\dot{V}O_2$ (51.4).

"wasted" ventilation, it is not surprising that a significantly higher ventilation is required for the same relative work among these patients.

ALVEOLAR-ARTERIAL PO₂ DIFFERENCE AND ARTERIAL END-TIDAL PCO₂ DIFFERENCE

In some patients, particularly those with pulmonary disease, it can be useful to quantify ventilation-perfusion inequality more directly. The alveolar-arterial PO_2 difference [$P(A-a)O_2$] is obtained by subtracting the arterial PO_2 (taken from an arterial blood gas sample) from the "ideal" alveolar PO_2. The ideal alveolar PO_2 is used because true alveolar PO_2 is usually impossible to obtain. The ideal alveolar PO_2 is that which the lungs would have if ventilation and perfusion were matched perfectly and if gas were exchanged at the same respiratory exchange ratio as in the real lungs. In normals, the alveolar-arterial PO_2 difference generally ranges from 10 to 15 mmHg at rest, and a slight widening tends to occur with exercise. When there is ventilation-perfusion inequality in the lung, the alveolar-arterial PO_2 difference tends to be larger, i.e., 30 to 40 mmHg or greater. This is commonly observed in patients with significant airway disease. In these patients, a reduced arterial PO_2 during exercise combined with increased cardiac output causes desaturated blood to flow through poorly ventilated areas of the lung.

When blood gases are available, the arterial end-tidal PCO_2 difference [P(a-ET)CO_2] can also provide evidence of elevated dead space or ventilation-perfusion mismatching. The arterial end-tidal PCO_2 difference is generally positive at rest (in the order of 1.0 to 5.0 mmHg) and decreases to below zero with exercise (-1.0 to -7.0 mmHg). When ventilation is high but perfusion is poor (such as in COPD), the value often remains positive with heavy exercise. When this occurs, V_D/V_T is often elevated and arterial oxygen saturation may fall.

BREATHING RESERVE

The **breathing reserve** is calculated as the ratio of maximal exercise ventilation to **maximal voluntary ventilation** at rest ($\dot{V}_E$ max/MVV). Most healthy subjects achieve a maximal ventilation of only 60% to 70% of MVV at peak exercise. One characteristic of chronic pulmonary disease is a maximal ventilation that approaches or equals the individual's MVV. These patients reach a "ventilatory" limit during exercise, while normal subjects generally have a substantial ventilatory reserve (20% to 40%) at peak exercise and are limited by other factors. A high breathing reserve is also usually observed in patients who are limited by cardiovascular disease (LV dysfunction or ischemia). Some debate exists as to how and whether MVV should be predicted, calculated directly, or determined from the **forced expiratory volume in one second (FEV$_1$)**. MVV is typically determined by breathing as rapidly, deeply, and forcefully as possible for either 12 or 15 sec and multiplying by 5 or 4, respectively. A reasonably accurate alternative is to multiply the FEV_1 by 40.

VENTILATORY THRESHOLD

The ventilatory or "anaerobic" threshold has a long history in exercise physiology. Because this issue continues to generate passionate debate, it warrants extended discussion. A physiological link between exercise capacity, lactate accumulation in the blood, and respiratory gas exchange was made by Hill and Lupton (17) more than 70 years ago. A sudden rise in the blood lactate level during exercise has long been associated with muscle anaerobiosis and has therefore been termed the "anaerobic threshold" (18). Historically, the anaerobic threshold has been defined as the highest oxygen uptake during exercise above which a sustained lactic acidosis occurs. When this level of exercise is reached, excess H^+ ions of lactate must be buffered to maintain physiological pH. Because bicarbonate buffering of lactate yields an additional source of CO_2 in the blood, ventilation is further stimulated. This point of nonlinear increase in ventilation has been used to detect the anaerobic threshold noninvasively and is often called the gas exchange anaerobic threshold (ATge) or the ventilatory threshold (VT) (Figure

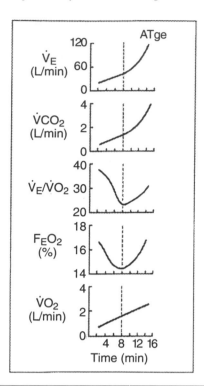

Figure 4.4   Gas exchange indices used to detect the ventilatory threshold (ATge). Reprinted from Froelicher et al. 1993.

4.4). Much confusion exists concerning the mechanism underlying this point and how it might be determined and applied clinically (19-21).

Changes in oxygen uptake at the VT have been used clinically during pharmacological and other investigations to imply that a change in oxygen supply to the working muscle has occurred. The anaerobic threshold has recently come under scrutiny, however, on both theoretical (20-21) and pragmatic (22-24) grounds. Connett et al. (25) studied dog gracilis muscle, which is a pure red fiber containing only type I and type IIA fibers, and observed lactate accumulation in those fibers under fully aerobic, mild (10% $\dot{V}O_2$max) conditions. These investigators also observed that lactate accumulation was not altered by changes in blood flow and that lactate accumulation occurred even though no anoxic areas were present in the muscle. This suggests that lactate production and muscle **hypoxia** are unrelated. Additionally, the advent of tracer technology has raised strong questions about the cause-and-effect relationship between oxygen availability to the muscle and the anaerobic threshold. Many studies now suggest that lactate production occurs at all times, even in resting conditions (21,25). Further, the turnover rate of lactate (the ratio of appearance and disappearance) is linearly related to oxygen uptake during exercise (20,26,27). This relationship is possible because recent studies have shown that lactate is "shuttled" from fibers where it is produced (presumably fast-twitch muscle) to those where it is used as an energy source (such as the heart and slow-twitch fibers). The "lactate shuttle" hypothesis has engendered the idea that production, transport, and use of lactate represents an important source of energy from carbohydrates during exercise (20,21).

Recent arguments have also been raised whether lactate in fact increases in a pattern that is mathematically "continuous" during exercise rather than as a threshold. Figure 4.5, a-b, illustrates two mathematical models that describe the relationship between lactate and oxygen uptake during exercise in one subject. In this subject, the "fit" for each model (determined by residual mean squared error) was about the same (28-31). The cumulative effect of these studies has led many to conclude that the "anaerobic" threshold is not related to muscle anaerobiosis but instead reflects simply an imbalance between lactate appearance and disappearance (20,21). When using gas exchange techniques, the term "ventilatory threshold" has been suggested as preferable to "anaerobic" as it does not imply the onset of anaerobiosis.

Lactate production and appearance in the blood during exercise appear to be related to several factors, including the rate of glycolytic flux, the isozyme form of lactate dehydrogenase (which catalyzes the conversion of pyruvate to lactate), as well as the availability of oxygen (32). The precise mechanism underlying the VT will continue to be argued. Irrespective of whether the VT is directly related to anaerobiosis, lactate does accumulate in the blood during exercise, ventilation must respond to maintain physiological pH, a breakpoint in ventilation appears to occur reproducibly (33), and this point is related to various measures of cardiopulmonary performance in normals (34-36) and patients with heart disease (18,37-41). A common argument in favor of the clinical use of the VT is that, as a submaximal parameter, it is better associated with patients' everyday activities than is maximal exercise, and using the VT avoids the increased risk and discomfort of maximal exercise.

From the many studies in this area, the following might be concluded:

- Regardless of the mechanism, ventilatory changes appear strongly correlated with a lactate threshold.
- An alteration in the VT reflects a change in the balance between lactate production and removal.
- References to muscle anaerobiosis should be avoided.

Lactate accumulation in the blood, and thus the VT, is associated with

- metabolic acidosis,
- hyperventilation,
- slowed oxygen uptake kinetics,
- accelerated glucose turnover,
- muscle fatigue, and
- a reduced capacity to perform work.

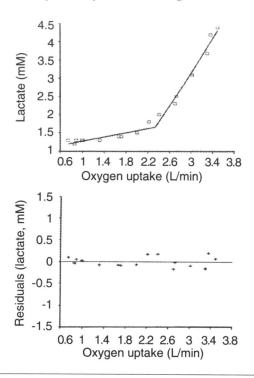

Figure 4.5a The relationship between lactate and oxygen uptake during exercise described using a log-log transformation model in which a threshold is represented by the intersection of two best fit lines to the data (mean squared error = 0.14) (26,28). Reprinted from Myers et al. 1994.

Therefore, a change in the lactate response to exercise that can be attributed to an intervention may add important information concerning the intervention. In this context, the VT during exercise testing remains an interesting and applicable index for use during exercise studies. However, the commonly used application of a given boundary (such as 40% or 50% $\dot{V}O_2$max) separating cardiovascular from pulmonary disorders requires further study.

An additional concern has been the method of choosing the VT. Our laboratory (24), along with others (22,23,42), has observed that the VT can vary markedly depending on the presence or absence of disease, method of determination, evaluator, and exercise protocol (Table 4.2 on p. 98). Although several methods of determination have been proposed, Caiozzo et al. (16) reported that the use of the ventilatory equivalents for oxygen ($\dot{V}_E/\dot{V}O_2$) and carbon dioxide ($\dot{V}_E/\dot{V}CO_2$) most closely reflected a lactate inflection point. Many laboratories have therefore defined the VT as the beginning of a systematic increase in $\dot{V}_E/\dot{V}O_2$ without a concomitant increase in $\dot{V}_E/\dot{V}CO_2$. However, methods of detecting the VT that rely on minute ventilation (such as the $\dot{V}_E/\dot{V}O_2$ method) may not be reliable under certain conditions (e.g., obesity, airflow obstruction, chemoreceptor

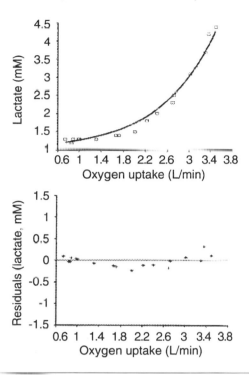

Figure 4.5b The relationship between lactate and oxygen uptake in the same subject as in Figure 4.5a during exercise described using a continuous exponential plus constant model (mean squared error = 0.008) (27). Reprinted from Myers et al. 1994

insensitivity) in which ventilation may lag behind metabolic events. Beaver et al. (43) therefore regressed $\dot{V}CO_2$ versus $\dot{V}O_2$ (called the **V-slope**) since carbon dioxide production more directly addresses lactate accumulation and is less influenced by noise or oscillatory changes in ventilation often noted in certain patients. These investigators reported that the detection of the VT was less difficult with the V-slope method.

In regard to interobserver agreement, we have successfully used a method outlined by Sullivan et al. (33) and modified by Shimizu et al. (24), in which two or more experienced, blinded (to patient name and test purpose, such as whether the test represents a drug or placebo phase) observers independently choose the VT for each exercise test. When a discrepancy exists, an additional observer is also blinded and chooses the VT independently. The VT is determined as the minute sample in which two of the three observers agree. The VT is not included in the analysis for that particular patient when all observers differ. Using 1-min samples of the ventilatory equivalents, we have found that out of three independent observers, two observers agree on 100% of exercise tests, and all three observers agree on 71% of the tests (33). In a more recent study, 7% of tests were excluded because all three observers disagreed (24). This technique

Table 4.2   Differences in Oxygen Uptake at the Ventilatory Threshold Due to Disease, Method of Determination, Evaluator, and Protocol

	% $\dot{V}O_2$max	$\dot{V}O_2$ (ml/min)
DISEASE		
Normal subjects ($n = 6$)	57.6 ± 14.3	1,469 ± 611
Patients ($n = 17$)	67.1 ± 10.6	937 ± 288
METHOD*		
$\dot{V}_E/\dot{V}O_2$	67.7 ± 12.7	1,128 ± 430
$P_{ET}O_2$	60.6 ± 13.6	1,003 ± 392
V-slope	65.4 ± 9.5	1,106 ± 482
EVALUATOR		
A	63.9 ± 11.3	1,067 ± 429
B	63.1 ± 12.7	1,048 ± 395
C	66.6 ± 13.1	1,118 ± 482
PROTOCOL		
Treadmill		
Bruce	68.2 ± 10.2	1,265 ± 417
Balke	68.9 ± 10.6	1,219 ± 486
Ramp	64.8 ± 13.4	1,107 ± 400
Bicycle		
25 W	61.3 ± 12.9	929 ± 390
50 W	62.7 ± 12.1	971 ± 368
Ramp	61.0 ± 13.0	964 ± 441

25 W = 25 watts/2-min stage; 50 W = 50 watts/2-min stage.

*$\dot{V}_E/\dot{V}O_2$ = the interval prior to the beginning of a systematic increase in the ventilatory equivalent for oxygen ($\dot{V}_E/\dot{V}O_2$) without an increase in the ventilatory equivalent for carbon dioxide. $P_{ET}O_2$ = the interval prior to the beginning of a systematic increase in the end-tidal pressure of oxygen ($P_{ET}O_2$) without a decrease in the end-tidal pressure of carbon dioxide. V-slope = the departure of $\dot{V}CO_2$ from a line of identity drawn through a plot of $\dot{V}CO_2$ versus $\dot{V}O_2$.

Modified from Shimizu et al. (24).

avoids interobserver bias and provides a means by which the VT can be determined objectively. Methods, problems, and advantages and disadvantages of various methods of choosing the VT or lactate inflection points have been the subjects of numerous reports (16,19-24,28-31,42-46).

Oxygen Uptake/Work Rate Relation

Many investigators have observed that patients with cardiovascular disease do not increase oxygen uptake as rapidly as normal subjects relative to the demands of the work (the work rate). Several laboratories have empirically quantified the relationship between increases in oxygen uptake and work rate, and they have compared the responses between normals and patients with cardiovascular or pulmonary disorders (47-52). These studies support the idea that oxygen uptake is limited by impaired oxygen delivery and that a reduction in the $\dot{V}O_2$/work rate relation can be a marker for cardiac dysfunction. However, the empirical approaches used, the many exercise protocols, and the well-known effects of beta-blockade on $\dot{V}O_2$ kinetics leave a considerable degree of confusion regarding how to apply this concept clinically. Hansen et al. (48) tested a group of normals and patients with various cardiovascular disorders on a cycle ergometer, and they expressed the $\dot{V}O_2$/work rate relation in terms of milliliters/minute increases in $\dot{V}O_2$ per increase in watts. Normal subjects exhibited a predictable increase of 10.16 ml/min/watt, whereas patients with cardiovascular or pulmonary disease demonstrated reduced responses ranging in the order of 7 to 8 ml/min/watt. We have evaluated normals and patients with cardiovascular disease in terms of the slope of the relationship between increases in work rate (expressed as predicted oxygen cost using ACSM equations) versus increases in measured oxygen uptake on various treadmill and cycle ergometer protocols (Figure 4.6) (49). Patients with chronic heart failure and coronary artery disease as well as those limited

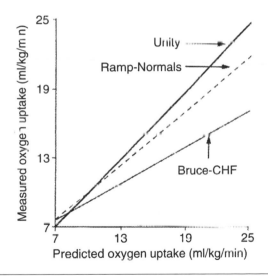

Figure 4.6 Relationship between the change in measured oxygen uptake and work rate (predicted oxygen uptake) among 10 normal subjects and 10 patients with chronic heart failure (CHF). The line of unity would be achieved if measured oxygen uptake increased in direct accordance with the change in work rate. Studies have shown that both the exercise protocol and the presence of disease can affect this relationship (in this case, the Ramp and Bruce treadmill protocols are compared). The slopes of these relationships were 0.53 for the patients and 0.81 for the normals. Reprinted from Myers et al. 1991.

by angina were found to have slope values that were significantly lower than those of normals (0.51 to 0.53 for the patients versus 0.81 for the normals). While these data (48,49) are consistent with others (47,50-54), many approaches and criteria have been used, and work is needed in this area to make this potentially valuable index more consistent for general application in the exercise laboratory.

Oxygen Kinetics

Although the measurement of oxygen kinetics often requires a specialized exercise test, is defined differently by various laboratories, and requires mathematical computations not familiar to most clinicians, this measurement is probably under-utilized as an index of cardiopulmonary function clinically. Like the $\dot{V}O_2$/work rate relation, oxygen kinetics quantify the ability of the cardiopulmonary system to respond to the demands of a given amount of work. It is frequently defined as the rate at which oxygen uptake reaches a steady-state value. However, measures such as the oxygen uptake/work rate relation, oxygen deficit, the steepness of the slope of the relationship between oxygen uptake and work rate (see Table 1.3 on p. 7), and various other measures of the difference between predicted and measured oxygen uptake generally describe oxygen kinetics. While mainly limited thus far to applications in human performance laboratories among healthy subjects, this is an untapped area for quantifying interventions in patients with heart disease.

A simplified model for estimating oxygen kinetics is illustrated in Figure 4.7. Models of oxygen kinetics have been used to study cardiovascular function before and after beta-blockade in which oxygen kinetics are slowed by propranolol and metoprolol (55-57). Hypoxia slows oxygen kinetics and causes a greater oxygen deficit and an increase in intramuscular lactate (58,59), whereas hyperoxia appears to enhance oxygen kinetics (58,59). Oxygen kinetics are greater below versus above the ventilatory threshold (60) and are greater after a program of physical conditioning (61). The implications of these findings for the study of pharmacologic interventions, exercise training, or other therapies in patients with heart or lung disease are intriguing, but few such studies have been done in the clinical setting.

Plateau in Oxygen Uptake

By defining the limits of the cardiopulmonary system, maximal oxygen uptake has been an invaluable measurement clinically for assessing a patient's clinical status, including the efficacy of drugs, exercise training, or invasive procedures. A question frequently raised is what exactly defines "maximal" oxygen uptake. From early studies using interrupted protocols, a test was only considered maximal when there was no further increase in oxygen uptake despite further increases in workload (i.e., a plateau). Conversely, oxygen uptake has been considered "peak" when the subject reaches a point of fatigue while no plateau in oxygen

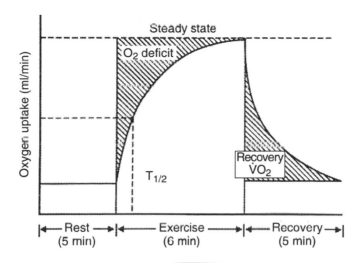

Figure 4.7 An example of a simplified model of a square-wave exercise test to determine oxygen uptake kinetics. The resting phase commonly consists of zero-load pedaling, steady state is some workload below the ventilatory threshold, and $T_{1/2}$ is the time required for a 50% change in oxygen uptake from rest to steady-state exercise. More complex models compute least-square fits or other mathematical functions through the exercise and recovery curves using breath-by-breath data.

uptake was observed. Unfortunately, the many problems associated with the determination and criteria for the plateau in oxygen uptake make these definitions more semantic than physiological. Because most exercise physiologists would probably consider this latter statement heretical, a brief history of the concept and its inherent problems is warranted.

In 1955, Taylor and associates (62) established the criteria of plateauing as a failure to increase oxygen uptake more than 150 ml/min, or 2.1 ml/kg/min with an increase in workload. This original research was performed using interrupted progressive treadmill protocols. With interrupted protocols, stages of exercise could be separated by rest periods ranging from minutes to days. Taylor and co-workers found that 75% of their subjects fulfilled these criteria. Using continuous treadmill protocols, Pollock et al. (63) found that 69%, 69%, 59%, and 80% of subjects plateaued when tested using the Balke, Bruce, Ellestad, and Åstrand protocols, respectively. Froelicher et al. (64) found that only 33%, 17%, and 7% of healthy aircrewmen met these criteria during testing with the Taylor, Balke, and Bruce protocols, respectively, although there were no significant differences between the protocols in maximal heart rate, $\dot{V}O_2$max, or maximal blood pressure. Taylor et al. later reported that plateauing generally did not occur when they used continuous treadmill protocols. More recent studies, using a variety of empirical criteria, report the occurrence of a plateau ranging from 7% to 90% of tests.

The plateau concept has been subjected to many interpretations and criteria. The newer, automated gas exchange systems that allow breath-by-breath or any specified sampling interval have raised new questions in regard to interpreting a plateau. Although the definitions of plateauing vary considerably, all focus on the idea that oxygen uptake at some point will fail to continue to rise as work increases. Using ramp treadmill testing in which work increases constantly at an individualized rate, we measured the slope of the change in work versus the change in oxygen uptake using different sampling intervals (65,66). In this way, if oxygen uptake were no longer increasing (while work increases continuously), the slope of the relationship between the two variables would not differ statistically from zero. To increase the possibility of observing a plateau, a large sampling interval of 30 consecutive eight-breath averages was used. Figure 4.8 illustrates the slope of each sample during the last several minutes of exercise in a healthy subject limited by fatigue. The open squares represent samples that had slopes significantly greater than zero (i.e., both work and oxygen uptake were increasing) and the closed squares represent samples that had slopes not different from, or less than, zero (i.e., work was increasing while oxygen uptake was not). This subject appeared to ''plateau'' at peak exercise. However, there also were several plateaus submaximally. Figure 4.9 illustrates the same subject using the same ramp protocol several days later. In this case, there were several plateaus submaximally, and no plateau was observed at peak exercise, although peak oxygen uptake and heart rate were the same. When the sampling interval was reduced

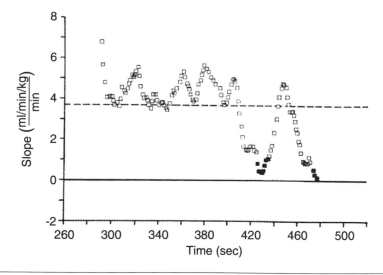

Figure 4.8 Individual slopes in oxygen uptake regressed with time for subject one on day one. Each darkened square represents a sample of 30 eight-breath averages in which the slope was not significantly greater than zero. Each open square denotes those that were greater than zero. The dashed line represents the mean of the observed change in oxygen uptake ([3.73 ml/kg/min]/min). Reprinted from Myers et al. 1989.

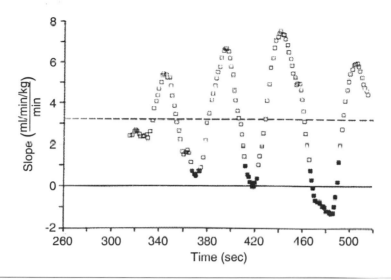

Figure 4.9 Individual slopes in oxygen uptake regressed with time for subject one on day two. Each darkened square represents a sample of 30 eight-breath averages in which the slope was not significantly greater than zero. Each open square denotes those that were greater than zero. The dashed line represents the mean of the observed change in oxygen uptake ([3.26 ml/kg/min]/min). Reprinted from Myers et al. 1989.

to 10 consecutive eight-breath averages, the variability was considerably greater. It appears that the slope of the change in oxygen uptake throughout progressive exercise varies greatly, despite a constant, consistent change in external work and the use of large, averaged samples. This degree of variability would appear to preclude the determination of a plateau by most definitions.

The plateau concept is long ingrained in exercise physiology. Intuitively, the body's respiratory and metabolic systems must reach some finite limit beyond which oxygen uptake can no longer increase, and some subjects who are highly motivated may exhibit a plateau. However, the occurrence of a plateau depends as much on the criteria applied, the sampling interval, and the methodology as the subject's health, fitness, and motivation. The demonstration of a plateau is unlikely to be crucial to clinical decision making. Recent data from our laboratory (65,66) and others (67,68) suggest that the plateau concept has limitations for general application during standard exercise testing.

SUMMARY

Gas exchange techniques provide a great deal of information about the capacity of the heart and lungs to delivery oxygen to the working muscle during exercise.

Maximal oxygen uptake defines the limits of the cardiopulmonary system; it is defined by cardiac output, by its redistribution during exercise, and by skeletal muscle metabolism. The combination of hemodynamic, gas exchange, and electro-cardiographic responses to exercise can be quite useful as a first step in quantifying the presence and extent of various cardiovascular and pulmonary disorders. These responses also help to guide therapy, make decisions regarding medical or surgical interventions, develop an exercise prescription, and stratify risk.

Since a primary responsibility of minute ventilation is to clear CO_2 from the blood, it is determined by both CO_2 production ($\dot{V}CO_2$) and arterial CO_2 pressure. The efficiency of ventilation is related to the ratio of air that participates in gas exchange (i.e., the alveolar ventilation), and that which does not (i.e., the dead space ventilation). The degree of dead space ventilation is important clinically, but its accurate measurement requires a direct determination of arterial CO_2 pressure. The ventilatory equivalents for oxygen ($\dot{V}_E/\dot{V}O_2$) and carbon dioxide ($\dot{V}_E/\dot{V}CO_2$) are also reflections of breathing efficiency, since they are influenced by the dead space ventilation. Even with maximal exercise, most healthy individuals have a substantial breathing reserve (the ratio of maximal ventilation during exercise to maximal voluntary ventilation at rest), suggesting the lungs normally do not limit exercise. When lactate accumulates in the blood during exercise of higher intensity, excess H^+ ions of lactate must be buffered to maintain physiological pH. The buffering process yields an additional source of CO_2, which further stimulates ventilation. This point has been called the ''ventilatory threshold.'' Despite significant disagreement over the mechanisms leading to lactate accumulation in the blood and how to define its ventilatory consequences, the ventilatory threshold maintains widespread application as a marker for cardiopulmonary performance both in the sport sciences and in clinical medicine.

In patients with pulmonary disease, more specialized measurements of ventilation-perfusion inequality are sometimes indicated. The alveolar-arterial PO_2 difference and the ventilatory dead space to tidal volume ratio require a direct measure of arterial blood gases. These indices more directly reflect ventilation-perfusion mismatching in the lungs. The oxygen uptake/work rate relation and measures of oxygen kinetics both reflect the capacity of the cardiopulmonary system to adapt to the demands of a given work rate.

Although a plateau in oxygen uptake has historically been considered a marker for maximal effort, it is often not observed clinically, and its utility has been limited by the many ways it has been defined and the differences in how gas exchange data are sampled.

REFERENCES

1. Zaret BL, Beller GA, eds. 1993. Nuclear Cardiology: State of the Art and Future Directions. St. Louis: Mosby-Year Book Medical.

2. Froelicher VF, Myers J, Follansbee WP, Labovitz AJ. 1993. Exercise and the Heart, 3d ed. St. Louis: Mosby-Year Book.

3. Marwick TH. 1994. Stress Echocardiography: Its Role in the Diagnosis and Evaluation of Coronary Artery Disease. Norwell, MA: Kluwer Academic.

4. Coyle EF, Martin WH, Ehsani AA, Hagberg JM. 1983. Blood lactate threshold in some well-trained ischemic heart disease patients. J Appl Physiol 54: 18-23.

5. Litchfield RL, Kerber RE, Benge JW, Mark AL, Sopko J, Bhatmagar RK, Marcus ML. 1982. Normal exercise capacity in patients with severe left ventricular dysfunction: Compensatory mechanisms. Circulation 66: 129-134.

6. Conley DL, Krahenbuhl GS. 1980. Running economy and distance running performance of highly trained athletes. Med Sci Sports Exerc 12: 357-360.

7. Pollock ML. 1977. Submaximal and maximal working capacity of elite distance runners. Part 1: Cardiorespiratory aspects. Ann NY Acad Sci 301: 310-321.

8. Ehsani AA, Hagberg JM, Hickson RC. 1978. Rapid changes in left ventricular dimensions and mass in response to physical conditioning and deconditioning. Am J Cardiol 42: 52-56.

9. Saltin B, Blomqvist G, Mitchell JH, Johnson RL Jr, Wilderthal K, Chapman CB. 1968. Response to exercise after bed rest and after training. Circulation 36 (suppl 7): 1-78

10. Blomqvist CG, Saltin B. 1983. Cardiovascular adaptations to physical training. Annu Rev Physiol 45: 169-189.

11. Ziesche S, Cobb FR, Cohn JN, Johnson G, Tristani F. 1993. Hydralazine and isosorbide diutrate combination improves exercise tolerance in heart failure. Results from V-Heft I and V-Heft II. Circulation 87 (suppl VI): VI-56–VI-64.

12. Morris CK, Ueshima K, Kawaguchi T, Hideg A, Froelicher VF. 1991. The prognostic value of exercise capacity: A review of the literature. Am Heart J 122: 1423-1431.

13. Mancini DM, Eisen H, Kussmaul W, Mull R, Edmunds LH, Wilson JR. 1991. Value of peak exercise oxygen consumption for optimal timing of cardiac transplantation in ambulatory patients with heart failure. Circulation 83: 778-786.

14. Vanhees L, Fagard R, Thijs L, Staessen J, Amery A. 1994. Prognostic significance of peak exercise capacity in patients with coronary artery disease. J Am Coll Cardiol 23: 358-363.

15. Nixon P, Orenstein DM, Kelsey SF, Doershuk CF. 1992. The prognostic value of exercise testing in patients with cystic fibrosis. N Engl J Med 327: 1785-1788.

16. Caiozzo VJ, Davis JA, Ellis JF, Azus JL, Vandagriff F, Prietto CA. 1982. A comparison of gas exchange indices used to detect the anaerobic threshold. J Appl Physiol 53: 1184-1189.

17. Hill AV, Lupton H. 1923. Muscular exercise, lactic acid, and the supply and utilization of oxygen. Q J Med 16: 135-171.
18. Wasserman K, McElroy MB. 1964. Detecting the threshold of anaerobic metabolism in cardiac patients during exercise. Am J Cardiol 14: 844-852.
19. Davis JA. 1985. Anaerobic threshold: Review of the concept and directions for future research. Med Sci Sports Exerc 17: 6-18.
20. Brooks GA. 1985. Anaerobic threshold: Review of the concept and directions for future research. Med Sci Sports Exerc 17: 22-31.
21. Brooks GA. 1986. Lactate production under fully aerobic conditions: The lactate shuttle during rest and exercise. Fed Proc 45: 2924-2929.
22. Gladden LB, Yates JW, Stremel RW, Stamford BA. 1985. Gas exchange and lactate anaerobic thresholds: Inter- and intra-evaluator agreement. J Appl Physiol 58: 2082-2089.
23. Yeh MP, Gardner RM, Adams TD, Yanowitz FG, Crapo RO. 1983. "Anaerobic threshold": Problems of determination and validation. J Appl Physiol 55: 1178-1186.
24. Shimizu M, Myers J, Buchanan N, Walsh D, Kraemer M, McAuley P, Froelicher VF. 1991. The ventilatory threshold: Method, protocol, and evaluator agreement. Am Heart J 122: 509-516.
25. Connett RJ, Gayeski TEJ, Honig GR. 1984. Lactate accumulation in fully aerobic working dog gracilis muscle. Am J Physiol 246: H120-H128.
26. Issekutz B, Shaw WAS, Issekutz AC. 1976. Lactate metabolism in resting and exercising dogs. J Appl Physiol 40: 312-319.
27. Stanley WC, Neese RA, Wisneski JA, Gertz EW. 1988. Lactate kinetics during submaximal exercise in humans: Studies with isotopic tracers. J Cardiopulmonary Rehabil 9: 331-340.
28. Beaver WL, Wasserman K, Whipp BJ. 1985. Improving detection of lactate threshold during exercise using a log-log transformation. J Appl Physiol 59: 1936-1940.
29. Hughson RL, Weisiger KH, Swanson GD. 1987. Blood lactate concentration increases as a continuous function during progressive exercise. J Appl Physiol 62: 1975-1981.
30. Myers J, Walsh D, Buchanan N, McAuley P, Bowes E, Froelicher VF. 1994. Increase in blood lactate during ramp exercise: Comparison of continuous versus threshold models. Med Sci Sports Exerc 26: 1413-1419.
31. Dennis SC, Noakes TD, Bosch AN. 1992. Ventilation and blood lactate increase exponentially during incremental exercise. J Sports Sci 10: 437-449.
32. Graham T. 1984. Mechanisms of blood lactate increase during exercise. Physiologist 27: 299.
33. Sullivan M, Genter F, Savvides M, Roberts M, Myers J, Froelicher VF. 1984. The reproducibility of hemodynamic, electrocardiographic, and gas exchange data during treadmill exercise in patients with stable angina pectoris. Chest 86: 375-381.
34. Davis JA, Frank MH, Whipp BJ, Wasserman K. 1979. Anaerobic threshold alterations caused by endurance training in middle-aged men. J Appl Physiol 46: 1039-1046.

35. Ready AE, Quinney HA. 1982. Alterations in anaerobic threshold as the result of endurance training and detraining. Med Sci Sports Exerc 14: 292-296.
36. Tanaka K, Matsura Y, Matsuzaka A, Hirakoba K. 1986. A longitudinal assessment of anaerobic threshold and distance running performance. Med Sci Sports Exerc 16: 278-282.
37. Sullivan MJ, Cobb FR. 1990. The anaerobic threshold in chronic heart failure: Relationship to blood lactate, ventilatory basis, reproducibility, and response to exercise training. Circulation 81: 1147-1158.
38. Matsumura N, Nishijima H, Kojima S, Hashimoto F, Minami M, Yasuda H. 1983. Determination of anaerobic threshold for assessment of functional state in patients with chronic heart failure. Circulation 68: 360-367.
39. Weber KT, Kinasewitz GT, Janicki JS, Fishman AP. 1982. Oxygen utilization and ventilation during exercise in patients with chronic cardiac failure. Circulation 65: 1213-1223.
40. Myers J, Atwood JE, Sullivan M, Forbes S, Friis R, Pewen W, Froelicher VF. 1987. Perceived exertion and gas exchange after calcium and beta-blockade in atrial fibrillation. J Appl Physiol 63: 97-104.
41. Sullivan M, Atwood AE, Myers J, Feuer J, Hall P, Kellerman B, Forbes S, Froelicher VF. 1989. Increased exercise capacity after digoxin administration in patients with heart failure. J Am Coll Cardiol 13: 1138-1143.
42. Dickstein K, Barvik S, Aarsland T, Snapinin S, Karlsson J. 1990. A comparison of methodologies in detection of the anaerobic threshold. Circulation 81 (suppl II): II-38–II-46.
43. Beaver WL, Wasserman K, Whipp BJ. 1986. A new method for detecting anaerobic threshold by gas exchange. J Appl Physiol 60: 2020-2027.
44. Hughes EF, Turner SC, Brooks GA. 1982. Effects of glycogen depletion and pedaling speed on "anaerobic threshold." J Appl Physiol 52: 1598-1607.
45. Whipp BJ, Ward SA, Wasserman K. 1986. Respiratory markers of the anaerobic threshold. Adv Cardiol 35: 47-64.
46. Gaesser GA, Poole DC. 1986. Lactate and ventilatory threshold: Disparity in time course of adaptations to training. J Appl Physiol 61: 999-1004.
47. Roberts JM, Sullivan M, Froelicher VF, Genter F, Myers J. 1984. Predicting oxygen uptake from treadmill testing in normal subjects and coronary artery disease patients. Am Heart J 108: 1454-1460.
48. Hansen JE, Sue DY, Oren A, Wasserman K. 1987. Relation of oxygen uptake to work rate in normal men and men with circulatory disorders. Am J Cardiol 59: 669-674.
49. Myers J, Buchanan N, Walsh D, Kraemer M, McAuley P, Hamilton-Wessler M, Froelicher VF. 1991. Comparison of the ramp versus standard exercise protocols. J Am Coll Cardiol 17: 1334-1342.
50. Auchincloss JH Jr, Ashutosh K, Rana S, Peppi D, Johnson LW, Gilbert R. 1976. Effect of cardiac, pulmonary, and vascular disease on one-minute oxygen uptake. Chest 70: 486-493.
51. Sullivan M, McKirnan MD. 1984. Errors in predicting functional capacity for post myocardial infarction patients using a modified Bruce protocol. Am Heart J 107: 486-492.

52. Solal AC, Chabernaud JM, Gourgon R. 1990. Comparison of oxygen uptake during bicycle exercise in patients with chronic heart failure and in normal subjects. J Am Coll Cardiol 16: 80-85.
53. Itoh H, Taniguchi K, Koike A, Doi M. 1990. Evaluation of severity of heart failure using ventilatory gas analysis. Circulation 81 (suppl II):II-31–II-37.
54. Tamesis B, Stelken A, Byers S, Shaw L, Younis L, Miller D, Chaitman BR. 1993. Comparison of the asymptomatic cardiac ischemia pilot and modified asymptomatic cardiac ischemia pilot versus Bruce and Cornell exercise protocols. Am J Cardiol 72: 715-720.
55. Hughson RL. 1984. Alterations in the oxygen deficit-oxygen debt relationships with beta-adrenergic receptor blockade in man. J Physiol (Lond.) 349: 375-387.
56. Petersen ES, Whipp BJ, Davis JA, Huntsman DJ, Brown HV, Wasserman K. 1983. Effects of beta-adrenergic blockade on ventilation and gas exchange during exercise in humans. J Appl Physiol 54: 1306-1313.
57. Twentyman OP, Disley A, Gribbin HR, Alberti KGM, Tattersfield AE. 1981. Effect of beta adrenergic blockade on respiratory and metabolic responses to exercise. J Appl Physiol 51: 788-792.
58. Linnarsson D. 1974. Dynamics of pulmonary gas exchange and heart rate changes at start and end of exercise. Acta Physiol Scand 415: 1-68.
59. Linnarsson D, Karlsson J, Fagraeus L, Saltin B. 1974. Muscle metabolites and oxygen deficit with exercise in hypoxia. J Appl Physiol 36: 399-402.
60. Sietsema KE, Daly JA, Wasserman K. 1989. Early dynamics of O_2 uptake and heart rate as affected exercise work rate. J Appl Physiol 67: 2535-2541.
61. Hickson RC, Bomze HA, Holloszy JO. 1978. Faster adjustment of O_2 uptake to the energy requirement of exercise in the trained state. J Appl Physiol 44: 877-881.
62. Taylor HL, Buskirk E, Heuschel A. 1955. Maximal oxygen intake as an objective measurement of cardiorespiratory performance. J Appl Physiol 8: 73-80.
63. Pollock ML, Bohannon RL, Cooper KH, Ayres JJ, Ward A, White SR, Linerud AC. 1976. A comparative analysis of four protocols for maximal treadmill stress testing. Am Heart J 92: 39-46.
64. Froelicher VF, Brammell H, Davis G, Noguera I, Stewart A, Lancaster MC. 1974. A comparison of the reproducibility and physiologic response to three maximal treadmill exercise protocols. Chest 65: 512-517.
65. Myers J, Walsh D, Buchanan N, Froelicher VF. 1989. Can maximal cardiopulmonary capacity be recognized by a plateau in oxygen uptake? Chest 96: 1312-1316.
66. Myers J, Walsh D, Sullivan M, Froelicher VF. 1990. Effect of sampling on variability and plateau in oxygen uptake. J Appl Physiol 68: 404-410.
67. Katch VL, Sady SS, Freedson P. 1982. Biological variability in maximum aerobic power. Med Sci Sports Exerc 14: 21-25.
68. Noakes TD. 1988. Implications of exercise testing for prediction of athletic performance: A contemporary perspective. Med Sci Sports Exerc 20: 319-330.

APPLICATIONS IN CARDIOVASCULAR AND PULMONARY DISEASE

*E*xercise testing can be used in various ways to evaluate patients with cardiovascular and pulmonary disorders. Aside from the most common application, diagnosis of coronary artery disease (CAD), the exercise test is used for assessing changes in symptoms, evaluating disability, and directing interventions such as bypass surgery, transplantation, or PTCA to the most appropriate patients. Because of the limitations in estimating exercise capacity from treadmill time and the greater yield of information from gas exchange analysis alluded to in earlier chapters, our bias has been to use gas exchange technology any time the test is performed for the purpose of addressing a research question.

Cardiopulmonary exercise testing does not by any means address all of the physician's clinical concerns about the patient. When performed properly, gas exchange techniques provide an accurate method of quantifying cardiopulmonary function. Few things, however, can replace the few moments the physician might spend before the test discussing the patient's history and performing a brief physical exam to determine the presence of edema, peripheral vascular disease, heart murmurs, and the like. A look at the resting 12-lead ECG can often tell much about the patient and may even contraindicate the test.

The exercise test is just one part of the patient workup; the addition of gas exchange techniques to the standard exercise test can yield more precise information about heart and lung function. It should be noted that any information gained from the test should be interpreted in the context of the patient's pretest characteristics and other responses known to contribute to diagnosis and prognosis. Gas exchange responses alone do not definitively confirm or deny the presence or absence of disease or establish prognosis.

The purpose of this chapter is to review some of these applications of cardiopulmonary exercise testing in cardiovascular and pulmonary disease. Because gas exchange analysis is a "graphic" technology, an effort is made to illustrate patient responses wherever possible. The following overview is not intended to be comprehensive, but it includes the major disorders that are commonly referred for exercise testing in our clinical and research laboratories.

CORONARY ARTERY DISEASE

Clinically, patients with coronary artery disease are the most common patients to be referred for an exercise test, and these patients are most often tested for the evaluation of chest pain (1). Although there has been a great deal of data reported among these patients using gas exchange analysis, most of it has been performed using small numbers of patients for research purposes, and it is not commonly used in the standard clinical setting. Exercise can be valuable in these patients because an imbalance between myocardial oxygen supply and demand (ischemia) is often not present at rest but manifests itself during exercise. For these patients the exercise test is a vital "gatekeeper" to more expensive and/ or invasive procedures. Expired gas analysis is not often needed if this is the test's only objective. However, it can be useful to note a number of differences in the gas exchange response between the patient with CAD and the normal individual (Table 5.1). When the patient's symptoms are mixed, precision is important, or it is unclear why the patient was referred, a cardiopulmonary test can be an important supplement to other clinical and exercise test information.

Relative to sedentary subjects of similar age, the hemodynamic response to exercise in CAD patients is characterized by reductions in maximal heart rate, systolic blood pressure, and cardiac output. There is a modest increase in filling pressure. At peak exercise, ejection fraction frequently decreases. Studies vary on the left ventricular volume response to maximal exercise in patients with coronary artery disease, but it appears that the volume response depends on the

Table 5.1   Common Responses to Exercise Testing in Coronary Artery Disease

- Reduced maximal oxygen uptake for age
- Chest pain
- Significant ST segment changes
- High breathing reserve
- Reduced oxygen uptake/work rate relation
- Steep heart rate/oxygen uptake relation
- Normal arterial O_2 saturation

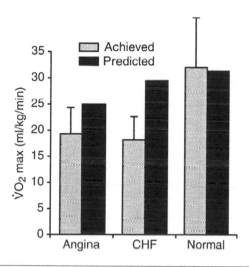

Figure 5.1   Achieved vs. age-predicted values for maximal oxygen uptake among patients with coronary artery disease limited by angina ($n = 16$), patients with chronic heart failure (CHF, $n = 40$), and normals ($n = 61$).

presence of symptoms, the ability to tolerate higher levels of exercise, and exercise position (2,3). During upright exercise, most studies have reported increases in both end-diastolic volume and end-systolic volume from rest to peak exercise in the order of 10% to 50% (3-7). Relative to normals, ventilatory gas exchange variables are reduced at peak exercise, particularly in patients limited by angina. It is common to observe maximal values that are roughly 60% to 70% of those achieved by normals among patients limited by angina (Figure 5.1). There also tends to be a low $\dot{V}O_2$ at the lactate or ventilatory threshold, a high breathing reserve (30% to 50%), an upward shift in the heart rate/oxygen uptake relationship (Figure 5.2)—with the notable exception of patients on beta-blockers—and a reduced slope of the relationship between $\dot{V}O_2$ and work rate.

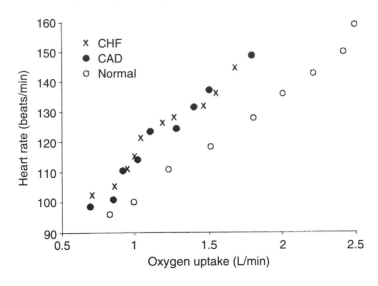

Figure 5.2   The relationship between heart rate and oxygen uptake in a group of patients with chronic heart failure (CHF, $n = 33$), a group of patients referred for PTCA (CAD, $n = 12$), and a group of sedentary normal subjects (normal, $n = 61$). Note the higher heart rate for any given oxygen uptake among the patients. Although there is a clear separation between patients and normals, it should be noted that there is considerable variability in the responses; the standard errors of the Y estimate for all three groups are in the order of 17 to 18 beats/min.

Ischemia can limit cardiac function, which can limit the increase in stroke volume (SV) and cardiac output. Anything that limits cardiac output will limit skeletal muscle perfusion, lead to fatigue, and therefore limit maximal oxygen uptake. A reduced capacity of the cardiopulmonary system to meet the demands dictated by the external workload underlies the reduction in the oxygen uptake/work rate relation; this can occur in any cardiovascular or pulmonary disease (8). This is particularly true at higher levels of work. The faster rise in heart rate relative to $\dot{V}O_2$ compared with normals suggests that increases in cardiac output rely more on increases in heart rate than stroke volume. In patients who have coronary artery disease that compromises ventricular function resulting in early metabolic acidosis, breathing patterns similar to those of patients with chronic heart failure can result, including high $\dot{V}_E/\dot{V}O_2$ and $\dot{V}_E/\dot{V}CO_2$ relationships and high V_D/V_T values.

CHRONIC HEART FAILURE

Patients with chronic heart failure (CHF) are a particularly interesting group because they exhibit so many abnormalities in ventilation and gas exchange

Table 5.2   Common Responses to Exercise Testing in Chronic Heart Failure

- Reduced maximal oxygen uptake for age
- High breathing reserve
- Normal arterial O_2 saturation
- Reduced oxygen uptake/work rate relation
- Steep heart rate/oxygen uptake relation
- Inefficient ventilation:
    High $\dot{V}_E/\dot{V}O_2$ and $\dot{V}_E/\dot{V}CO_2$
    High V_D/V_T
- Chronotropic incompetence
- Attenuated blood pressure response

during exercise (Table 5.2). Clinically, the severity of heart failure is often classified in terms of the degree of **dyspnea** or fatigue in response to various levels of exertion. Exercise intolerance secondary to severe CHF can be disabling, even to the point where it can prohibit activities of daily living. A striking characteristic of the exercise response in CHF is relative hyperventilation. Many laboratories in recent years have demonstrated markedly elevated ventilatory responses among patients with CHF compared with normal subjects at similar work rates (9-13).

Historically, the mechanism for the hyperventilatory response to exercise in these patients has focused on increased intrapulmonary pressures, which are related to interstitial fluid accumulation, decreased lung compliance (14-16), and stimulation of pulmonary juxtacapillary receptors in the lungs (15,17,18). It has been thought that these receptors, which are stimulated by distension of the pulmonary vessels, are the primary cause of dyspnea in CHF. However, direct evidence of a link between elevated intrapulmonary pressures and dyspnea during exercise is lacking (11,19-21), and the physiologic mechanism that underlies exertional hyperventilation in patients with CHF remains unclear (9,22). Several other mechanisms have been proposed to account for exertional hyperventilation in these patients.

Early metabolic acidosis has been observed by several investigators (10,12,23-27). Weber et al., for example, reported that mixed venous lactate levels were higher for the same absolute workload as the severity of CHF increased (12). Because lactate buffering yields an additional source of CO_2 in the blood, ventilation is stimulated. Other investigators (9,10,27) have observed higher V_D/V_T values at rest and during exercise among CHF patients versus normals, suggesting that larger areas of the lung are present with poor ventilation-perfusion ratios, causing a greater degree of ventilation to be wasted. Although the possibility of altered ventilatory control mechanisms has been raised (17,28), Sullivan et al. (9) recently reported that arterial PCO_2 and the ratio of alveolar ventilation to

$\dot{V}CO_2$ were maintained during exercise, which suggests that neural and chemo-receptor control mechanisms were intact in patients with CHF.

The greater ventilatory requirement for any given oxygen uptake is evidenced by the data shown in Figure 5.3. The ventilatory equivalents for oxygen ($\dot{V}_E/\dot{V}O_2$) were approximately 25% to 30% higher at matched relative work intensities throughout exercise among patients with CHF compared with normal subjects of similar age. One contributor to inefficient ventilation in patients with CHF is illustrated in Figure 5.4: patients with CHF generally demonstrate poor exercise capacity and a large fraction of dead space (V_D/V_T). Because anatomic dead space is generally related to length of the conducting airways, it should not be different among adults, and the differences between normals and CHF patients are most likely due to physiologic dead space. An elevated V_D/V_T, which suggests a ventilation-perfusion mismatch in the lungs, is an important factor governing the ventilatory requirement for work in CHF patients. An improvement in ventilation-perfusion matching, which could be accomplished either by an increase in cardiac output or a reduction in physiologic dead space, has the potential for improving exercise capacity in these patients.

It was recently observed that an improvement in exercise capacity after digoxin administration was associated with an improved V_D/V_T (29). Sullivan et al. (9) studied 64 patients with chronic CHF, and in addition to an elevated V_D/V_T compared with that of normal subjects, they reported an inverse relationship between maximal ventilation and maximal cardiac output and a direct relationship between maximal ventilation and maximal V_D/V_T. These data suggest that

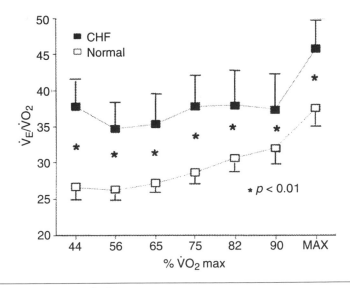

Figure 5.3   Changes in $\dot{V}_E/\dot{V}O_2$ expressed as a percentage of maximal oxygen uptake for patients with CHF and normal subjects (mean ± 2 SEM). Reprinted from Myers et al. 1992.

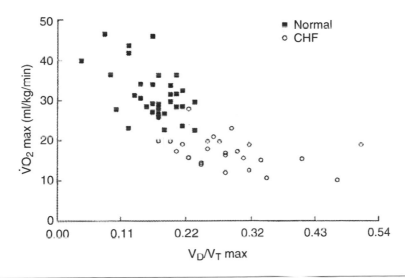

Figure 5.4   The relationship between maximal ventilatory dead space to tidal volume ratio (V_D/V_T max) and maximal oxygen uptake ($\dot{V}O_2$max) for normal subjects (■) and patients with chronic heart failure (○). The correlation coefficient between the two variables was −0.73 (standard error of estimate = 6.2; $p < 0.001$). Reprinted from Myers et al. 1992.

ventilation-perfusion abnormalities in CHF patients are closely linked to both poor cardiac output and underperfused areas in the lung. It follows that a reduction in V_D/V_T would occur concomitantly with an increase in pulmonary blood flow as a result of an improvement in cardiac output.

A final notable characteristic of the patient with chronic heart failure that also contributes to inefficient ventilation is an abnormal breathing pattern. Figure 5.5 compares V_D/V_T, respiratory rate, and tidal volume at matched levels of exercise between patients with heart failure and normals. In normal subjects, a marked reduction in V_D/V_T occurs as exercise progresses; in contrast, only minimal change occurs among CHF patients. The higher V_D/V_T in CHF patients could be caused by either an elevated physiologic dead space or a reduction in tidal volume. In an effort to compensate for large amount of physiologic dead space in these patients, respiratory rate increases, while the depth of breathing remains shallow. This abnormal and inefficient breathing pattern in CHF is accentuated at maximal exercise. In spite of the fact that mean maximal ventilation was roughly 36 L/min lower in patients with CHF, respiratory rate was slightly higher, tidal volume was roughly 30% lower, and V_D/V_T was nearly twice that of normal subjects.

At low levels of exercise, most of the differences in V_D/V_T between groups were attributable to a greater degree of physiologic dead space. As exercise progressed, the reduced tidal volume made a greater contribution to V_D/V_T, even though at maximal exercise, most of the differences between groups were attributable to an increased amount of dead space. The high respiratory rate is

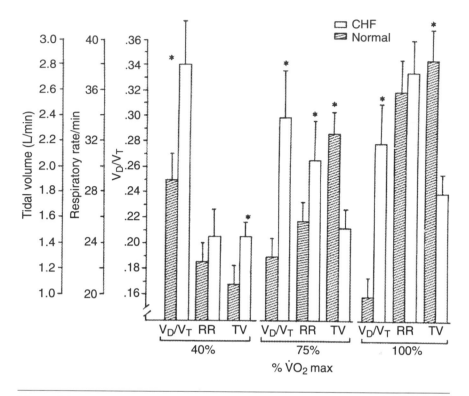

Figure 5.5   Mean (± 2 SEM) values for V_D/V_T, respiratory rate (RR), and tidal volume (TV) at matched percentages of maximal oxygen uptake among patients with CHF and normal subjects ($p < 0.01$). Reprinted from Myers et al. 1992.

needed to compensate for both the elevation in dead space and the reduction in tidal volume. However, the mechanism that underlies the shallow tidal volume in these patients is unknown. Because pulmonary hemodynamics are abnormal, the lungs are less compliant and the work of breathing is increased in patients with CHF. Thus, a common explanation given for the peculiar breathing pattern in these patients is the reduced work of breathing associated with more rapid but shallow respiration (15).

PULMONARY DISEASE

In normal individuals, the argument is often made that $\dot{V}O_2$max is limited by the heart and not the lungs or periphery. A characteristic of the patient with pulmonary disease is that the lungs limit exercise. There is little, if any, breathing reserve, and the inability to adequately ventilate the alveoli during exercise leads to a drop in arterial oxygen saturation. Chronic pulmonary diseases that can limit exercise generally fall into two categories: those affecting the pulmonary vasculature, and those involving a primary airflow obstruction. The pulmonary vasculature may be the site of an intrinsic disorder, or there may be secondary involvement of the pulmonary vasculature due to congestive heart failure, valvular disease, or congenital heart disease. Causes of primary pulmonary vascular disease include thromboemboli, intrapulmonary shunt, and pulmonary hypertension. Obstructive lung diseases include **emphysema**, chronic bronchitis, asthma, and combinations of these. Any of these conditions may significantly alter lung mechanics and/or impair gas exchange, lead to dyspnea, and reduce exercise tolerance.

Patients with pulmonary disease become dyspneic with low or modest levels of activity. Dyspnea reflects the balance between ventilation necessary for metabolism and the patient's capacity to transfer air into and out of the lungs. The ratio of maximum $\dot{V}_E$ to MVV is usually quite high (close to 100%), particularly in patients with chronic airflow obstruction. In general, this contrasts the 30% to 50% breathing reserve found in most normals and patients with heart disease. A decrease in arterial oxygen saturation is a hallmark of pulmonary disease. This is due to increases in pulmonary vascular resistance, pulmonary hypertension, and a reduction in the alveolar surface area for diffusion. Abnormal diffusion capacity is exacerbated during exercise, since pulmonary blood flow is greater and pulmonary capillary transit time is faster.

In patients with chronic bronchitis or asthma, airway resistance is increased, which reduces ventilatory capacity. In emphysema, marked airflow obstruction and reduced elastic recoil combine to reduce ventilatory capacity. In both cases, an increase in the ventilatory requirement occurs because of the mismatching of ventilation to perfusion, making ventilation highly inefficient. Gas exchange data will exhibit high V_D/V_T values, i.e., there will be greater "wasted" ventilation for each breath. This will also be reflected by higher than normal ventilatory equivalents for oxygen and CO_2 ($\dot{V}_E/\dot{V}O_2$ and $\dot{V}_E/\dot{V}CO_2$). As with any condition that hinders the capacity to ventilate, exchange, or deliver oxygen to the working muscle, the $\dot{V}O_2$/work rate relation is reduced in patients with pulmonary disease (Table 5.3).

Table 5.3   Common Responses to Exercise Testing in Pulmonary Disease

- Reduced maximal oxygen uptake for age
- Reduced breathing reserve ($\dot{V}_E$ max/MVV)
- Rapid, shallow respiration
- Inefficient ventilation (high V_D/V_T, $\dot{V}_E/\dot{V}O_2$, $\dot{V}_E/\dot{V}CO_2$)
- Arterial oxygen desaturation
- Reduced oxygen uptake/work rate relation
- Elevated arterial end-tidal PCO_2 difference

VALVULAR DISEASE

Efficient delivery of blood to the tissues requires healthy, functioning valves to ensure the movement of blood in one direction. Heart valves can either become stenotic (i.e., they do not open completely), impeding the flow of blood, or leak (they do not close properly, i.e., become insufficient or regurgitant), such that some portion of blood is pumped backward. Both can lead to a major hemodynamic burden. Valvular stenosis leads to a ''pressure overload'' of the chamber proximal to the diseased valve, and a regurgitant valve leads to a ''volume overload'' by the chamber involved. The reduction in exercise capacity is related to the severity of the stenosis or regurgitation and to which valve is involved.

Valvular heart disease has been listed as a ''relative'' contraindication to exercise testing in the American Heart Association and American College of Sports Medicine guidelines (30,31). Severe aortic stenosis is an absolute contraindication; effort syncope in these patients is an important and well-appreciated symptom, and there have been reports of cardiac arrest (32). However, several large trials have reported that event rates in patients with valvular disease are extremely low when the test is performed with appropriate supervision (32). The exercise test can play an important role in the objective assessment of symptoms, hemodynamic responses, and functional capacity. By performing exercise testing preoperatively and postoperatively, one can quantify baseline impairment and the benefits of surgery. Exercise testing offers the opportunity to evaluate objectively any disparities between history and clinical findings, for example, in the elderly ''asymptomatic subject'' with physical or Doppler findings of severe aortic stenosis. Often, echocardiographic studies are inadequate in such patients, particularly among smokers. When Doppler echocardiography reveals a significant gradient in the asymptomatic patient with normal exercise capacity, he or she could be followed closely until symptoms develop. In patients with an inadequate rise in systolic blood pressure or when a fall in systolic pressure occurs concomitantly with symptoms, surgery is often indicated.

Maximal oxygen uptake is reduced considerably in patients with valvular disease (32-34). Few data are available using gas exchange analysis in patients with valvular disease. There are limited data to justify the concept that, like patients with end-stage heart failure who are selected for transplant, patients with valvular disease who do not achieve a peak $\dot{V}O_2$ greater than 14 to 15 ml/kg/min stand to benefit the most from valve replacement. Based on the survival data reported among patients with severe chronic heart failure, several laboratories use this or similar criteria to help select patients for valve replacement, but there are not yet enough data to make such a universal recommendation.

Valvular disease underlies the symptoms associated with many patients who have atrial fibrillation or chronic heart failure. In mitral stenosis, heart rate is generally higher during exercise to compensate for a reduced stroke volume, but cardiac output remains low relative to oxygen uptake (14). The characteristic inefficient ventilation and rapid, shallow respiration often seen in patients with heart failure have been observed in patients with mitral stenosis (14,17,34,35). Naturally, any impediment to mitral flow will lead to higher than normal pulmonary pressures and reduced pulmonary compliance, and such observations have been documented in these patients (14,36,37). These factors will increase the dead space fraction of ventilation. Mitral valve replacement and valvulotomy have been shown to reduce pulmonary vascular resistance and improve the ventilatory response to exercise (17,38). In aortic stenosis, chamber dilatation and myocardial hypertrophy compensate such that exercise capacity is generally higher than in mitral stenosis; cardiac output and maximal oxygen uptake are compromised only in severe aortic stenosis. Maximal exercise testing in patients with aortic stenosis may require particular precautions, including frequent monitoring of blood pressure and rhythm (32).

ATRIAL FIBRILLATION

The major hemodynamic characteristic of atrial fibrillation is an irregular, often rapid, ventricular rate at rest and during exercise. An uncontrolled ventricular response is generally thought to hinder cardiac performance during exercise due to a compromised cardiac output, consistent with a lack of atrial contribution to ventricular filling and a shortened ventricular filling time (39-41). This is thought by some investigators to account for the reduced exercise tolerance observed among patients with atrial fibrillation compared with normals (42-46). However, whether the uncontrolled heart rate responses themselves are responsible for the attenuation of exercise tolerance in these patients is unclear (45,47). Hornsten and Bruce (48), for example, reported that despite an increase in submaximal and maximal heart rates of roughly 25 beats/min among patients with atrial fibrillation compared with age-matched normals, exercise capacity was not different between groups.

Atwood and associates (45) studied the exercise response of 50 patients with atrial fibrillation using gas exchange techniques and reported elevations in heart rate at rest and during exercise that were similar to previous studies. Interestingly, although patients with lone atrial fibrillation (atrial fibrillation without apparent underlying disease) achieved maximal oxygen uptake values that were similar to those expected for age, patients with atrial fibrillation and underlying heart disease (valvular, ischemic, or cardiomyopathic) had significantly reduced exercise capacity. Thus, it appears that the exercise impairment in chronic atrial fibrillation reported by some investigators is due to underlying heart disease and not the arrhythmia itself.

Using resting echocardiography and gas exchange techniques during exercise, Ueshima et al. (47) recently made detailed studies of 79 patients with chronic atrial fibrillation. They divided patients by history into lone (atrial fibrillation without underlying heart disease), hypertensive, heart failure, ischemia, and valvular heart disease groups. Maximal ventricular rates were markedly elevated except in patients with a history of heart failure or valvular disease, who achieved heart rates typical of those expected for normal subjects of similar age. While left atrial dimensions were elevated for all groups (45 to 55 mm), left ventricular ejection fractions were normal (58% to 59%) for all but the heart failure group (44.6%). Both systolic and diastolic ventricular dimensions were normal for all groups. Using multiple regression techniques, maximal oxygen uptake was poorly explained by left ventricular morphology and function. Among hemodynamic variables, only maximal systolic pressure and maximal heart rate were significant predictors of maximal oxygen uptake; 45% of the variance in maximal oxygen uptake was accounted for by these two variables. Maximal oxygen uptake was reduced only in the heart failure and valvular disease groups, but maximal heart rates were 25 to 30 beats lower in these patients also, suggesting reduced cardiac outputs. These data appear to confirm that the major clinical concern for atrial fibrillation is the "company it keeps." The arrhythmia itself does not underlie any major hemodynamic compromise.

Four groups of investigators have employed gas exchange techniques to evaluate the effect of electrical conversion to sinus rhythm on the response to exercise among patients with atrial fibrillation (46,49-51). These studies generally demonstrated modest (roughly 10% to 20%) improvements in maximal oxygen uptake after conversion to normal sinus rhythm, confirming the general clinical impression that an appropriately timed atrial systole makes modest contributions to ventricular filling and therefore increases stroke volume and cardiac output (39-48). Lipkin et al. (49) reported no improvement in maximal oxygen uptake and echocardiographic variables one day after successful cardioversion, but significant improvements in stroke volume and maximal oxygen uptake were observed a month later. The delayed improvement in exercise capacity is provocative, given that a similar delay is commonly observed despite immediate hemodynamic improvements following pharmacologic treatment in patients with chronic heart failure (22). Atwood and associates (46) reported a significant improvement in maximal oxygen uptake after successful cardioversion, but a mean 48 beats/min reduction in maximal heart rate left many patients chronotropically incompetent after the procedure. These investigators observed that the relationship between ventilation and carbon dioxide production changed after cardioversion (Figure 5.6). Ventilation was reduced for any given carbon dioxide production at higher levels of exercise, suggesting a modest improvement in the efficiency of ventilation. This increase in efficiency occurred to a degree that paralleled the improvement in maximal oxygen uptake. These observations were confirmed in a more recent study by Lundstrom and Karlsson (51), who also documented a concomitant increase in cardiac output, suggesting that an improvement in the matching of ventilation to perfusion in the lungs underlies the improvement in ventilatory efficiency.

CARDIAC TRANSPLANTATION

Over the last two decades, transplantation has become a widely used and successful treatment option for patients with end-stage heart failure. In 1990, the 1-year

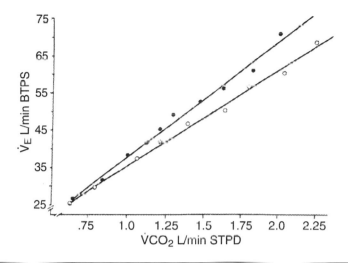

Figure 5.6 The relationship between minute ventilation and CO_2 production pre (●) and post (○) cardioversion to normal sinus rhythm. Note the slightly more efficient ventilation while in normal sinus rhythm, which paralleled the improvement in $\dot{V}O_2$max. Reprinted from Atwood et al. 1989.

and 5-year survival rates for this procedure were reported to be 81% and 72%, respectively (52). The hemodynamic response to exercise in patients who have undergone cardiac transplantation has been characterized since the early 1970s (53-55). Because the heart is denervated, some intriguing hemodynamic responses are observed. Orthotopic transplantation removes the nervous system connections to the heart. Thus, the heart is not responsive to the normal actions of the parasympathetic and sympathetic systems. The absence of vagal tone explains the high resting heart rates in these patients (100 to 110 beats/min) and the relatively slow adaptation of the heart to a given amount of submaximal work (53). This slows the delivery of oxygen to the working tissue, contributing to an earlier than normal metabolic acidosis and hyperventilation during exercise (54-58). Maximal heart rate is lower in transplant patients compared with normals, which contributes to a reduction in cardiac output and $\dot{V}O_2$max; a-vO_2 difference widens as a compensatory mechanism. Higher than normal increases in the ventilatory equivalents for oxygen and carbon dioxide are observed. These increases are attributable to uneven matching of ventilation to perfusion and an increase in physiologic dead space. Lower than normal end-diastolic volumes have been observed in transplant patients, and filling pressures are inordinately high during supine exercise, suggesting reduced compliance (59-62).

Is transplantation effective in improving the gas exchange response to exercise in patients with end-stage heart failure? Several groups have addressed this issue in recent years. Central hemodynamics at rest and during exercise, including pulmonary capillary wedge pressure, right atrial pressure, and cardiac index (CI) show marked improvements 1 year after transplantation (63). Marzo et al. (57) recently reported a 39% increase in $\dot{V}O_2$max 1 year after transplantation, along with a delay in the ventilatory threshold (22% increase in $\dot{V}O_2$). Submaximal ventilation and the ventilatory equivalents for oxygen and carbon dioxide were also improved after transplantation. However, the ventilatory response to exercise remained excessive relative to normals. Warner-Stevenson et al. (64) reported similar improvements in $\dot{V}O_2$max and $\dot{V}O_2$ at the ventilatory threshold between patients who underwent transplantation and those who survived more than 6 months on sustained medical therapy. These studies underscore the important fact that transplantation does not restore a normal hemodynamic and ventilatory response to exercise and that surgery patients should be carefully selected. The latter group of investigators have employed the precision offered by gas exchange analysis to help optimize the selection of patients for transplantation (65). Patients on a waiting list who improved maximal $\dot{V}O_2$ and $\dot{V}O_2$ at the ventilatory threshold by small degrees (greater than 2 ml/kg/min) were removed from the list, and no deaths were observed after a mean of 18 months of follow-up. Mancini et al. (66) reported marked differences in survival between patients on a transplant waiting list who achieved a peak $\dot{V}O_2$ of $\geq$ 14 ml/kg/min and those $\leq$ 14 ml/kg/min. The 1-year survival rate of patients with the higher peak $\dot{V}O_2$ values was similar to those who received transplantation (94%), whereas those with the lower peak $\dot{V}O_2$ had a 1-year survival rate of 47%.

Table 5.4 presents mean responses to maximal exercise performed in stable patients 6 months to 3 years after undergoing transplantation at Stanford University. Note the limited exercise capacity relative to age, the blunted heart rate and systolic blood pressure responses, and the highly inefficient ventilatory response, with ventilatory equivalents for oxygen and carbon dioxide of 55.0 and 41.3, respectively, at peak exercise. Numerous factors, of course, contribute to these patients' abnormal response to exercise before and after transplantation, and one wouldn't expect a transplanted heart alone to completely normalize ventilatory responses. Pulmonary function is highly abnormal among patients awaiting transplantation, which can be attributed to cardiomegaly, interstitial edema, and pleural effusion (67). At least one study has noted marked improvements in **forced vital capacity (FVC)** and FEV_1 values after transplantation (67). Naturally, patients with end-stage disease are highly deconditioned, which contributes to a wide range of central and peripheral abnormalities in response to exercise (22).

CARDIAC PACEMAKERS

Implantable pacemakers are devices designed to compensate for abnormalities in the heart's electrical conduction system. Today, pacemakers range from simple, single-chamber, fixed-rate devices to complex, dual-chamber instruments (a pacing lead in both the atrium and ventricle) that "sense" physiologic information to stimulate the heart's electrical activity, essentially substituting for the sinus

Table 5.4   Responses to Symptom-Limited Cardiopulmonary Exercise Testing in 20 Stable Patients (Age = 50 ± 11) 6 Months to 3 Years Following Cardiac Transplantation

Variable	Rest	Ventilatory threshold	Peak exercise	% predicted
Heart rate (beats/min)	90 ± 22	120 ± 23	141 + 31	83
Systolic blood pressure (mmHg)	107 ± 15	122 ± 20	144 ± 31	
Diastolic blood pressure (mmHg)	71 ± 9	68 ± 8	75 ± 8	
Work (watts)	0	73 ± 30	112 ± 62	46.3
Oxygen uptake (ml/kg/min)	4.4	10.1 ± 4	15.5 ± 5	48.7
CO_2 production (L/min)	0.227	1.080 ± 0.610	1.650 ± 1.08	
Respiratory exchange ratio	0.76	0.91 ± 0.12	1.19 ± 0.12	
Respiratory rate (breaths/min)	16	23.0 ± 6	34.9 ± 8.6	
Tidal volume (ml)	701	1289 ± 460	1954 ± 1014	
V_D/V_T	0.36	0.35 ± 0.08	0.24 ± 0.08	
O_2 pulse (ml/beat)	2.8	5.5 ± 3	10.6 ± 5	
Ventilation (L/min)	11.2	29.7 ± 16	68.2 ± 23	49.0
$\dot{V}_E/\dot{V}O_2$	31.8 ± 7	36.7 ± 9	55.0 ± 14	
$\dot{V}_E/\dot{V}CO_2$	49.3 ± 11	27.5 ± 9	41.3 ± 11	

node. Sensors detect changes in body motion or activity, the flow of electrical current, body chemistry, temperature, or pressure. Combined with dual-chamber technology and proper programming, these sensors can virtually duplicate the normal heart's chamber synchrony and chronotropic function.

The different types of pacemakers and sensors have advantages and disadvantages (68,69). Differences in daily activity levels can make a particular sensor better for some patients than for others. The concept that pacemakers can automatically adjust their rates based on the sensing of variables that correlate with oxygen uptake has led to an abundance of studies using gas exchange techniques in the last decade. Choosing the appropriate type of pacemaker and programming it properly for a given patient can present a challenge, and gas exchange information during exercise is routinely used by some laboratories to optimize pacemaker information. Because heart rate is the most important factor governing cardiac output during exercise (and thus oxygen uptake), appropriate pacing is particularly important among patients who continue to work, participate in rehabilitation, or lead an active lifestyle.

Naturally, an increase in peak oxygen uptake through an improvement in rate responsiveness is important to document, and gas exchange techniques have been used to accurately assess exercise capacity in patients after pacemaker

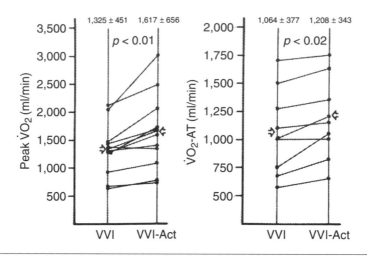

Figure 5.7 Comparison of oxygen uptake values in 12 patients at peak exercise and the ventilatory threshold ($\dot{V}O_2$-AT), using fixed rate pacing (VVI) versus a pacing system that adjusts the pacing rate by tracking physical activity (VVI-Act). The unfilled arrows indicate the mean values. Reprinted from Benditt et al. 1987.

implantation and to follow them serially (Figure 5.7). However, investigators have been even more interested in the pattern of the gas exchange response to exercise. While varying pacemaker sensing devices, atrial rates, or ventricular rates, researchers have assessed oxygen kinetics, alterations in the ventilatory threshold, ventilatory efficiency, the effect of rate responsive pacing on differences between measured and predicted oxygen uptake, and the relation between changes in ventricular rates and oxygen uptake or work during exercise (70-77). As pacemaker technology continues to evolve, gas exchange techniques will no doubt play an integral part in assessing maximum benefit to the patient.

SUMMARY

Gas exchange techniques have many applications among patients with cardiovascular and pulmonary disease. Recent studies suggest that the added precision provided by this technology has important prognostic utility. A cardiopulmonary exercise test can supplement other clinical and exercise test information when precision is important, the patient's symptoms are mixed, or it is unclear why the patient was referred for testing. Patients with either cardiovascular or pulmonary disease often have substantially reduced values for maximal oxygen uptake compared with normals. Both the patient with coronary artery disease and the patient with chronic heart failure generally exhibit a normal breathing reserve and a normal arterial oxygen saturation. The patient with chronic heart failure, however, frequently breathes inefficiently during exercise, as evidenced by higher than normal ventilatory equivalents for $\dot{V}O_2$ and $\dot{V}CO_2$. These abnormal gas exchange responses are due to the combination of a mismatching of ventilation and perfusion in the lungs and early metabolic acidosis.

In addition to similar inefficient ventilatory patterns, patients with pulmonary disease generally exhibit a reduced breathing reserve and often demonstrate arterial oxygen desaturation. Exercise limitation results from an abnormally increased ventilatory requirement while ventilatory capacity is reduced. Data have been published concerning breathing patterns, breathing efficiency, oxygen kinetics, and blood gas responses to exercise that characterize the response to exercise among transplant recipients and patients with atrial fibrillation, valvular disease, and pacemakers. Two studies performed among patients with chronic atrial fibrillation recently demonstrated an improvement in the efficiency of ventilation after electrical conversion to sinus rhythm. Interest has been generated in the 1990s regarding the gas exchange response to exercise among pre- and postcardiac transplant patients. Gas exchange abnormalities in end-stage chronic heart failure are significantly improved by transplantation, and studies have shown that the gas exchange response of transplant candidates helps to optimize the selection of patients for transplantation.

REFERENCES

1. Miranda CP, Lehmann KG, Froelicher VF. 1989. Indications, criteria for interpretation, and utilization of exercise testing in patients with coronary artery disease: Results of a survey. J Cardiopulmonary Rehabil 9: 479-484.
2. Froelicher VF, Myers J, Follansbee WP, Labovitz AJ. 1993. Exercise and the Heart, 3d ed. St. Louis: Mosby-Year Book.
3. Manyeri DE, Kostuk WJ. 1983. Right and left ventricular function at rest and during bicycle exercise in the supine and sitting positions in normal subjects and patients with coronary artery disease. Assessment by radionuclide ventriculography. Am J Cardiol 51: 36-42.
4. Rerych SK, Scholz PM, Newman GE, Sabiston DC Jr, Jones RH. 1978. Cardiac function at rest and during exercise in normals and in patients with coronary heart disease. Evaluation by radionuclide angiography. Ann Surg 187: 449-464.
5. Freeman MR, Berman DS, Staniloff H, El Kayam V, Maddahi J, Swan HJC, Forrester J. 1981. Comparison of upright and supine bicycle exercise in the detection and evaluation of extent of coronary artery disease by equilibrium radionuclide ventriculography. Am Heart J 102: 182-189.
6. Shen WF, Roubin GS, Choong CY-P, Hutton BF, Harris PJ, Gletcher PJ, Kelley DT. 1985. Left ventricular response to exercise in coronary artery disease: Relation to myocardial ischemia and effects of nifedipine. Eur Heart J 6: 1025-1031.

7. Kalisher AL, Johnson LL, Johnson YE, Stone J, Feder JL, Escala E, Cannon PJ. 1984. Effects of propranolol and timolol on left ventricular volumes during exercise in patients with coronary artery disease. J Am Coll Cardiol 3: 210-218.

8. Hansen JE, Sue DY, Oren A, Wasserman K. 1987. Relation of oxygen uptake to work rate in normal men and men with circulatory disorders. Am J Cardiol 59: 669-674.

9. Sullivan MJ, Higginbotham MB, Cobb FR. 1988. Increased exercise ventilation in patients with chronic heart failure: Intact ventilatory control despite hemodynamic and pulmonary abnormalities. Circulation 77: 552-559.

10. Roubin GS, Anderson SD, Shen WF, Choong CY-P, Alwyn M, Hillery S, Harris PJ, Kelley DT. 1990. Hemodynamic and metabolic basis of impaired exercise tolerance in patients with severe left ventricular dysfunction. J Am Coll Cardiol 15: 986-994.

11. Fink LI, Wilson JR, Ferraro N. 1986. Exercise ventilation and pulmonary artery wedge pressure in chronic stable congestive heart failure. Am J Cardiol 57: 249-253.

12. Weber KT, Kinasewitz GT, Janicki JS, Fishman AP. 1982. Oxygen utilization and ventilation during exercise in patients with chronic cardiac failure. Circulation 65: 1213-1223.

13. Rubin SA, Brown HV. 1984. Ventilation and gas exchange during exercise in severe chronic heart failure. Am Rev Respir Dis 129 (suppl): 563-564.

14. Gazetopolous N, Davies H, Oliver C, Deuchan D. 1966. Ventilation and hemodynamics in heart disease. Br Heart J 28: 11-16.

15. Ingram RH, McFadden ER. 1976. Respiratory changes during exercise in patients with pulmonary venous hypertension. Prog Cardiovasc Dis 19: 109-115.

16. Parker GW, Gorlin R. 1969. Immediate post-exercise vital capacity: A measure of increased pulmonary capillary pressure. Am J Med Sci 257: 365-370.

17. Reed JW, Ablett M, Cotes JE. 1978. Ventilatory responses to exercise and to carbon dioxide in mitral stenosis before and after valvulotomy: Causes of tachypnoea. Clin Sci Molecular Med 54: 9-16.

18. Paintal AS. 1969. Mechanism of stimulation of type J pulmonary receptors. J Physiol 203: 511-532.

19. Szlachcic J, Massie BM, Kramer BL, Topic N, Tubau J. 1985. Correlates of prognostic implication of exercise capacity in chronic congestive heart failure. Am J Cardiol 55: 1037-1042.

20. Wilson JR, Ferraro N. 1983. Exercise intolerance in patients with chronic left heart failure: Relation to oxygen transport and ventilatory abnormalities. Am J Cardiol 51: 1358-1363.

21. Lipkin DP, Canepa-Anson R, Stephens MR, Poole-Wilson PA. 1986. Factors determining symptoms in heart failure: Comparison of fast and slow exercise tests. Br Heart J 55: 439-445.

22. Myers J, Froelicher VF. 1991. Hemodynamic determinants of exercise capacity in chronic heart failure. Ann Intern Med 115: 377-386.

23. Reddy HK, Weber KT, Janicki JS, McElroy PA. 1988. Light isometric exercise in patients with chronic cardiac failure. J Am Coll Cardiol 12: 353-358.
24. Cowley AJ, Stainer K, Rowley JM, Hampton JR. 1986. Abnormalities of the peripheral circulation and respiratory function in patients with severe heart failure. Br Heart J 55: 75-80.
25. Sullivan MJ, Higginbotham MB, Cobb FR. 1989. Exercise training in patients with chronic heart failure delays ventilatory anaerobic threshold and improves submaximal exercise performance. Circulation 79: 324-329.
26. Weber KT, Janicki JS. 1985. Lactate production during maximal and submaximal exercise in patients with chronic heart failure. J Am Coll Cardiol 6: 717-724.
27. Myers J, Salleh A, Buchanan N, Smith D, Neutel J, Bowes E, Froelicher VF. 1992. Ventilatory mechanisms of exercise intolerance in chronic heart failure. Am Heart J 124: 710-719.
28. Oren A, Wasserman K, Davis JA, Whipp BJ. 1981. Effect of CO_2 set point on ventilatory response to exercise. J Appl Physiol 51: 185-189.
29. Sullivan M, Atwood JE, Myers J, Feuer J, Hall P, Kellerman B, Forbes S, Froelicher VF. 1989. Increased exercise capacity after digoxin administration in patients with heart failure. J Am Coll Cardiol 13: 1138-1143.
30. Fletcher GF, Balady G, Froelicher VF, Hartley LH, Haskell WL, Pollock ML. 1995. Exercise standards: A statement for health professionals from the American Heart Association. Circulation 91: 580-615.
31. American College of Sports Medicine. 1995. Guidelines for Exercise Testing and Exercise Prescription, 5th ed. Philadelphia: Lea and Febiger.
32. Atwood JE, Kawanishi S, Myers J, Froelicher VF. 1988. Exercise testing in patients with aortic stenosis. Chest 93: 1083-1087.
33. Chapman CB, Mitchell JH, Sproule BJ, Potter D, Williams B. 1960. The maximal oxygen intake test in patients with predominant mitral stenosis. Circulation 22: 4-13.
34. Blackmon JR, Rowell LB, Kennedy JW, Twiss RD, Conn RD. 1967. Physiological significance of maximal oxygen intake in "pure" mitral stenosis. Circulation 36: 497-510.
35. Nery LE, Wasserman K, French W, Oren A, Davis JA. 1983. Contrasting cardiovascular and respiratory responses to exercise in mitral valve and chronic obstructive pulmonary diseases. Chest 83: 446-453.
36. Carstens V, Behrenbeck DW, Hilger HH. 1983. Exercise capacity before and after cardiac valve surgery. Cardiology 70: 41-49.
37. Saxton GA, Robinowitz M, Dexter L, Haynes F. 1956. The relationship of pulmonary compliance to pulmonary vascular pressures in patients with heart disease. J Clin Invest 35: 611-618.
38. Zener JC, Hancock EW, Shumway NE, Harrison DC. 1972. Regression of extreme pulmonary hypertension after mitral valve surgery. Am J Cardiol 30: 820-826.

39. Braunwald E. 1964. Symposium on cardiac arrhythmias: Introduction with comments on the hemodynamic significance of atrial systole. Am J Med 37: 665-669.

40. Skinner NS, Mitchell JH, Wallace AG, Sarnoff SJ. 1964. Hemodynamic consequences of atrial fibrillation at constant ventricular rates. Am J Med 36: 342-351.

41. Samet P, Bernstein W, Levine S. 1965. Significance of the atrial contribution to ventricular filling. Am J Cardiol 15: 195-202.

42. Orlando JR, Van Herick R, Aronow WS, Olson HG. 1979. Hemodynamics and echocardiograms before and after cardioversion of atrial fibrillation to normal sinus rhythm. Chest 76: 521-526.

43. Morris JJ, Entman M, North WC, Kong Y, McIntosh H. 1965. The changes in cardiac output with reversion of atrial fibrillation to sinus rhythm. Circulation 31: 670-678.

44. Shapiro W, Klein G. 1968. Alterations in cardiac function immediately following electrical conversion of atrial fibrillation to normal sinus rhythm. Circulation 38: 1074-1084.

45. Atwood JE, Myers J, Sullivan M, Forbes S, Friis R, Pewen W, Callaham P, Hall P, Froelicher V. 1988. Maximal exercise testing and gas exchange in patients with chronic atrial fibrillation. J Am Coll Cardiol 11: 508-513.

46. Atwood JE, Myers J, Sullivan M, Forbes S, Sandhu S, Callaham P, Froelicher VF. 1989. The effect of cardioversion on maximal exercise capacity in patients with chronic atrial fibrillation. Am Heart J 118: 913-918.

47. Ueshima K, Myers J, Ribisl PM, Atwood JE, Morris CK, Kawaguchi T, Liu J, Froelicher VF. 1993. Hemodynamic determinants of exercise capacity in chronic atrial fibrillation. Am Heart J 125: 1301-1305.

48. Hornsten TR, Bruce RA. 1968. Effects of atrial fibrillation on exercise performance in patients with cardiac disease. Circulation 37: 543-548.

49. Lipkin DP, Fremeauz M, Stewart R, Joshi J, Lowe T, McKenna WJ. 1988. Delayed improvement in exercise capacity after cardioversion of atrial fibrillation to sinus rhythm. Br Heart J 59: 572-577.

50. Ueshima K, Myers J, Morris CK, Atwood JE, Kawaguchi T, Froelicher VF. 1993. The effect of cardioversion on exercise capacity in patients with atrial fibrillation. Am Heart J 126: 1021-1024.

51. Lundstrom T, Karlsson O. 1992. Improved ventilatory response to exercise after cardioversion of chronic atrial fibrillation to sinus rhythm. Chest 102: 1017-1022.

52. Kriett JM, Kaye MP. 1990. The registry of the International Society for Heart Transplantation: Seventh official report—1990. J Heart Transplant 9: 323-330.

53. Stinson EB, Griepp RL, Schroeder JS, Dong E, Shumway NE. 1972. Hemodynamic observations one and two years after cardiac transplantation in man. Circulation 14: 1181-1193.

54. Savin W, Haskell WL, Schroeder JS, Stinson EB. 1980. Cardiorespiratory responses of cardiac transplant patients to graded, symptom-limited exercise. Circulation 62: 55-60.

55. Schroeder JS. 1979. Hemodynamic performance of the human transplanted heart. Transplant Proc 11: 304-308.
56. Degre SGL, Niset GL, De Smet JM, Ibrahim T, Stoupel E, et al. 1987. Cardiorespiratory response to early exercise testing after orthotopic cardiac transplantation. Am J Cardiol 60: 926-928.
57. Marzo KP, Wilson JR, Mancini DM. 1992. Effects of cardiac transplantation on ventilatory response to exercise. Am J Cardiol 69: 547-553.
58. Brubaker PH, Berry MJ, Brozena SC, Morley DL, Walter JD, Paolone AM, Bove AA. 1993. Relationship of lactate and ventilatory thresholds in cardiac transplant patients. Med Sci Sports Exerc 25: 191-196.
59. Hosenpud JD, Morton MJ, Wilson RA, Pantely GA, Norman DJ, Cobanoglu MA, Starr A. 1989. Abnormal exercise hemodynamics in cardiac allograft recipients one year after cardiac transplantation: Relation to preload reserve. Circulation 80: 525-532.
60. Pflugfelder PW, Purves PD, McKenzie FN, Kostuk WJ. 1987. Cardiac dynamics during supine exercise in cyclosporine-treated orthotopic heart transplant recipients: Assessment by radionuclide angiography. J Am Coll Cardiol 10: 336-341.
61. Pflugfelder PW, McKenzie FN, Kostuk WJ. 1988. Hemodynamic profiles at rest and during supine exercise after orthotopic cardiac transplantation. Am J Cardiol 61: 1328-1333.
62. Pflugfelder PW, Purves PD, Menkis AH, McKenzie FN, Kostuk WJ. 1989. Rest and exercise left ventricular ejection and filling characteristics following orthotopic cardiac transplantation. Can J Cardiol 5:161-167.
63. Rudas L, Pflugfelder PW, McKenzie FN, Menkis AH, Novick RJ, Kostuk WJ. 1992. Normalization of upright exercise hemodynamics and improved exercise capacity one year after orthotopic cardiac transplantation. Am J Cardiol 69: 1336-1339.
64. Warner-Stevenson L, Sietsma K, Tillisch JH, Lem V, Walden J, Kobashigawa JA, Moriguchi J. 1990. Exercise capacity for survivors of cardiac transplantation or sustained medical therapy for stable heart failure. Circulation 81: 78-85.
65. Warner-Stevenson L, Stiemle AE, Chelimsky-Fallick C, Hamilton MA, Moriguchi JD, Kermani M, Lem V, Tillisch JH. 1992. Ability to improve exercise capacity identifies heart transplant candidates who should leave the waiting list. Circulation 86 (suppl I): I-809.
66. Mancini DM, Eisen H, Kussmaul W, Mull R, Edmunds LH, Wilson JR. 1991. Value of peak exercise oxygen consumption for optimal timing of cardiac transplantation in ambulatory patients with heart failure. Circulation 83: 778-786.
67. Hosenspud J, Stibolt T, Atwal K, Shelley D. 1990. Abnormal pulmonary function specifically related to congestive heart failure: Comparison of patients before and after cardiac transplantation. Am J Med 88: 493-496.
68. Kristensson B, et al. 1985. The haemodynamic importance of atrioventricular synchrony and rate increase at rest and during exercise. Eur Heart J 6: 668-673.

69. Lau CP, Butrous GS, Ward DE, Camm AJ. 1989. Comparison of exercise performance of six rate-adaptative right ventricular cardiac pacemakers. Am J Cardiol 63 (12): 833-888.
70. French WJ, Haskell RJ, Wesley GW, Florio J. 1988. Physiological benefits of a pacemaker with dual chamber pacing at low heart rates and single chamber rate responsive pacing during exercise. Pace 11: 1840-1845.
71. Vogt P, Goy JJ, Kuhn M, Leuenberger P, Kappenberger L. 1988. Single versus double chamber rate responsive cardiac pacing: Comparison by cardiopulmonary noninvasive exercise testing. Pace 11: 1896-1901.
72. Benditt DG, Milstein S, Buetikofer J, Gornick CC, Mianulli M, Fetter J. 1987. Sensor-triggered, rate-variable cardiac pacing. Ann Intern Med 107: 714-724.
73. Rossi P, Rognoni G, Occhetta E, Aina F, Prando MD, Plicchi G, Minella M. 1985. Respiration-dependent ventricular pacing compared with fixed ventricular and atrial-ventricular synchronous pacing: Aerobic and hemodynamic variables. J Am Coll Cardiol 6: 646-652.
74. Casaburi R, Spitzer S, Wasserman K. 1989. Effect of altering heart rate on oxygen uptake at exercise onset. Chest 95: 6-12.
75. Benditt DG, Mianulli M, Fetter J, Benson DW, Dunnigan A, Molina E, Gornick CC, Almquist A. 1987. Single-chamber cardiac pacing with activity-initiated chronotropic response: Evaluation by cardiopulmonary exercise testing. Circulation 75: 184-191.
76. Haskell RJ, French WJ. 1989. Physiological importance of different atrioventricular intervals to improved exercise performance in patients with dual chamber pacemakers. Br Heart J 61: 46-51.
77. McElroy PA, Janicki JS, Weber KT. 1988. Physiologic correlates of the heart rate response to upright isotonic exercise: Relevance to rate-responsive pacemakers. J Am Coll Cardiol 11: 94-99.

NORMAL VALUES FOR EXERCISE CAPACITY

*I*t is well known that maximal oxygen uptake declines with increasing age and that higher values are observed in men. Thus, when measuring or estimating maximal oxygen uptake, it is useful to have reference values for comparison. Many investigators have developed reference values for measured maximal oxygen uptake adjusted for age and gender, and the reader is referred to these sources for more detail (1-9). However, determining what constitutes "normal" can be an arduous undertaking. Although numerous descriptive studies have been performed in this area, few of the population samples have been large enough to firmly establish "normal standards," and all are specific to the population from which they are drawn. In addition, the data are rather sparse in terms of normal standards for variables other than maximal oxygen uptake, such as maximal ventilation, V_D/V_T, breathing frequency, and end-tidal pressures. The purpose of this chapter is to provide an overview of what has been published concerning predicted values for exercise capacity. The major considerations include the factors that influence the prediction of exercise capacity, the limitations involved, the units by which one expresses "normal," the many regression equations that have been developed, and the application of nomograms.

FACTORS AFFECTING REFERENCE VALUES FOR EXERCISE CAPACITY

Many clever attempts have been made to improve the prediction of what represents a "normal" exercise capacity by including height, weight, body composition, activity status, exercise mode, and such clinical and demographic factors as smoking history, heart disease, and medications. It is important to note that a "normal" value is only a number that has been inferred from some population. A predicted normal value usually refers to age and gender, but many other factors affect one's exercise capacity. In addition to those mentioned above, these include some that are not so easily measured, such as genetics and the type and extent of disease. In the classic studies of Bruce and associates (4), gender and age were the most important factors influencing exercise capacity (compared with activity status, weight, height, or smoking). This has since been confirmed by our laboratory (10) and others (11). However, the relation between age and exercise capacity is highly imprecise. Figure 6.1 illustrates the relationship between maximal oxygen uptake and age, with different levels of current physical activity considered (12). The wide scatter around the regression lines and poor correlation coefficients underscore the common observation that a great deal of inaccuracy exists when we attempt to predict exercise capacity from age, even when considering other factors such as gender or activity level. Choosing the most appropriate reference equation is therefore critical. Table 6.1 (p. 134) outlines the various factors to consider where applying reference formulas.

UNITS FOR EXPRESSION OF NORMAL

The energy cost of work can be expressed in absolute oxygen uptake, oxygen uptake relative to body weight, METs, kilocalories, watts, and other units. When discussing normal values, it is important to consider how they are expressed. Because the mass of the exercising muscle is greater in a heavier individual, the energy cost of any submaximal activity is greater, and it is often assumed that maximal oxygen uptake would be greater since body dimensions should determine the maximal quantity of oxygen that can be delivered. It is important to note, however, that oxygen uptake is related to the exercising muscle mass, not to total weight or adipose tissue. Indeed, studies have shown that body weight per se does not strongly influence $\dot{V}O_2max$ (3,11,15). Correlations between exercise

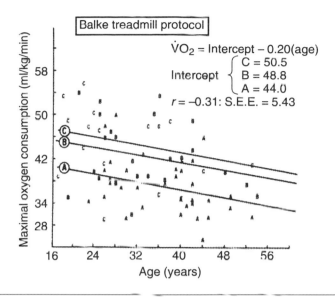

Figure 6.1   Relationship between maximal oxygen uptake and age among 79 men with current physical activity status considered. A = sedentary, B = moderate exercisers, C = heavy exercisers, SEE = standard error of the estimate. Reprinted from Froelicher et al. 1975.

capacity and body composition, expressed as percent body fat or body mass index, have ranged widely from $r = -0.15$ to -0.66 (10,13,14). A more important consideration is the units by which exercise capacity is expressed. Because $\dot{V}O_2$ in ml/kg/min normalizes exercise capacity for body weight, weight-bearing activities such as treadmill walking are usually expressed by these "relative" units. The commonly used clinical expression, METs, is simply a multiple of the $\dot{V}O_2$ in ml/kg/min at rest (assumed to be 3.5 ml/kg/min).

REGRESSION EQUATIONS

The following are commonly used generalized equations based on data published in North America and Europe in the 1950s, 1960s, and 1970s (5-8):

Males

$$\dot{V}O_2max \ (L/min) = 4.2 - 0.032 \ (age) \ (SD \pm 0.4)$$

$$\dot{V}O_2max \ (ml/kg/min) = 60 - 0.55 \ (age) \ (SD \pm 7.5)$$

Females

$$\dot{V}O_2max \ (L/min) = 2.6 - 0.014 \ (age) \ (SD \pm 0.4)$$

$$\dot{V}O_2max \ (ml/kg/min) = 48 - 0.37 \ (age) \ (SD \pm 7.0)$$

Table 6.1   Factors to Consider in Reference Population When Applying Formulas for Exercise Capacity

- Population tested:
  - Age
  - Gender
  - Anthropometric characteristics
  - Health and fitness
  - Heart disease
  - Pulmonary disease
- Exercise mode and protocol
- Reason tested:
  - Clinical referral
  - Screening apparently healthy volunteers
- Exercise capacity estimated versus measured directly
- Units of measurement
- Variability of predicted values (usually 10% to 30%)

Note that for middle-aged individuals, the variability for these predicted values is roughly 20%.

Efforts have been made to improve the precision of predictive equations by considering specific populations, body size, and other demographic factors, in addition to gender. Hansen et al. (3) and Wasserman et al. (2) have published predicted values for measured oxygen uptake that consider sex, age, height, weight, and whether testing was performed on a treadmill or a cycle ergometer:

	Mode	Over-weight	Predicted $\dot{V}O_2$max (ml/min)
Males	Cycle*	No	Wt $\times$ [50.72 $-$ (0.372 $\times$ A)]
		Yes	[0.79 $\times$ (Ht $-$ 60.7)] $\times$ [50.72 $-$ (0.372 $\times$ A)]
	Treadmill**	No	Wt $\times$ [56.36 $-$ (0.413 $\times$ A)]
		Yes	[0.79 $\times$ (Ht $-$ 60.7)] $\times$ [56.36 $-$ (0.413 $\times$ A)]
Females	Cycle*	No	(42.8 $\times$ Wt) $\times$ [22.78 $-$ (0.17 $\times$ A)]
		Yes	Ht $\times$ [14.81 $-$ (0.11 $\times$ A)]
	Treadmill***	No	Wt $\times$ [44.37 $-$ (0.413 $\times$ A)]
		Yes	[0.79 $\times$ (Ht $-$ 68.2)] $\times$ [44.37 $-$ (0.413 $\times$ A)]

Wt = weight in kg; Ht = height in cm; A = age in years
  *Overweight is Wt > [0.79 $\times$ (Ht $-$ 60.7)].
 **Overweight is Wt > [0.65 $\times$ (Ht $-$ 42.8)].
***Overweight is Wt > [0.79 $\times$ (Ht $-$ 68.2)].

Jones et al. (16) studied healthy adults on a cycle ergometer and reported the following regression equation:

$$\dot{V}O_2max \ (L/min) = 0.046(Ht) - 0.021(age) - 0.62(gender) - 4.31$$
$$(r = 0.87, SEE = 0.46)$$

Ht = height in cm, and gender is coded 0 for males, 1 for females

Although normal values had been derived from Scandinavian children in the 1950s (17), Cooper and Weiler-Ravell (18) more recently developed regression equations from California school children (ages 6 to 17) that considered height rather than age:

$$Boys: \dot{V}O_2 \ (ml/min) = 43.6(Ht) - 4547$$
$$Girls: \dot{V}O_2 \ (ml/min) = 22.5(Ht) - 1837$$

Ht = height in cm

APPLICATION OF NOMOGRAMS

Unfortunately, few clinical exercise laboratories measure oxygen uptake directly, and various methods have been developed using estimated values from exercise times or workloads achieved. One of the early techniques was developed by Bruce et al. (4), who suggested the use of a nomogram for estimating **functional aerobic impairment (FAI)** (Figure 6.2). In this nomogram, one side depicts treadmill time using the Bruce protocol and the other side depicts age. Between these two lines are percent increments of FAI for sedentary and active individuals. By drawing a straight line through age (from which maximal oxygen uptake can be predicted) and the treadmill time, an estimate of aerobic impairment can be read from the sloped lines. A "normal" value would be zero, since observed exercise capacity should be the same as that predicted. The problem with this approach is, of course, that relatively poor correlations between age and maximal oxygen uptake have been demonstrated in healthy and diseased individuals even when activity levels are considered (Figure 6.1). Many factors affect an individual's aerobic capacity besides current activity level, including

- past activity level,
- genetic endowment,
- mechanical efficiency,
- previous testing experience, and
- specificity of training.

Thus, this nomogram was based on two poor relationships, which thereby limit its ability to predict functional capacity.

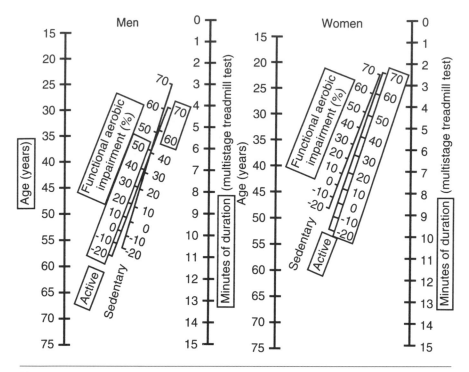

Figure 6.2 Nomograms for healthy middle-aged men (left) and women (right) for determining percent deviation from normal values for exercise capacity among active and sedentary individuals. "Minutes of duration" refers to treadmill time on the Bruce protocol, and a negative number represents a fitter-than-average response. Reprinted from Bruce, Kusumi, and Hosmer 1973.

Morris and associates (9) recently developed a similar nomogram from 1,388 male patients. This nomogram is of interest clinically because it is based on METs achieved from treadmill speed and grade and does not restrict one to using the Bruce protocol, and it was derived from a group of males who were referred for exercise testing for clinical reasons. The regression equations derived from the group were

$$\text{All subjects: METs} = 18.0 - 0.15(\text{age})$$
$$\text{SEE} = 3.3, r = -0.46, p < 0.001$$
$$\text{Active subjects: METs} = 18.7 - 0.15(\text{age})$$
$$\text{SEE} = 3.0, r = -0.49, p < 0.001$$
$$\text{Sedentary subjects: METs} = 16.6 - 0.16(\text{age})$$
$$\text{SEE} = 3.2, r = -0.43, p < 0.001$$

These nomograms are illustrated in Figures 6.3 and 6.4. Such nomograms are advantageous because they offer a simple visual method of assessing a patient's

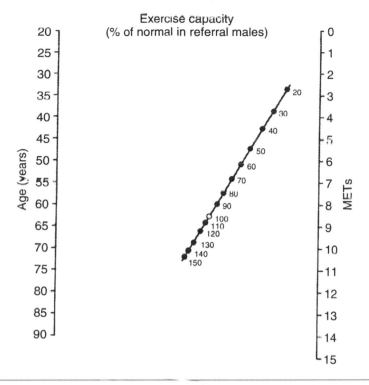

Figure 6.3 Nomogram of percent normal exercise capacity for age in 1,388 male veterans referred for exercise testing (based on metabolic equivalents [METs]). Reprinted from Morris et al. 1993.

response relative to his or her peers, while avoiding having to make cumbersome calculations from a particular regression equation. However, when using regression equations or nomograms for reference purposes, it is important to consider several points. First, as mentioned, the relationship between exercise capacity and age is rather poor ($r = -0.30$ to -0.60). Second, nearly all equations are derived from different populations using different protocols; thus, they are both population and protocol specific. For example, the equations developed by Morris et al. (9) were derived from a large group of veterans referred for testing for clinical reasons. They had a higher prevalence of heart disease than that found in most other studies, and it is not surprising that a greater slope was present with a faster decline in $\dot{V}O_2max$ with age. In addition, since treadmill time or workload tends to overpredict maximal METs, it is important to consider whether gas exchange techniques were used in developing the equations.

To account for the differences due to measured versus predicted oxygen uptake and those due to the presence of disease, Morris et al. (9) also developed a nomogram using measured oxygen uptake among 244 active or sedentary apparently healthy males (Figures 6.5 on p. 139 and 6.6 on p. 140). The MET values

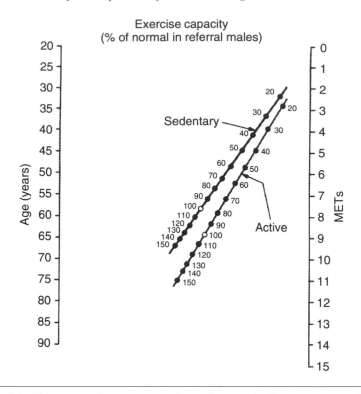

Figure 6.4   Nomogram of percent normal exercise capacity for age among active (*n* = 346) and sedentary (*n* = 253) males referred for exercise testing. METs = metabolic equivalents. Reprinted from Morris et al. 1993.

are shifted downward roughly 1.0 to 1.5 METs for any given age, reflecting the lower but more precise measures of exercise capacity.

$$\text{All subjects: METs} = 14.7 - 0.11(\text{age})$$
$$\text{SEE} = 2.5, r = -0.53, p < 0.001$$
$$\text{Active subjects: METs} = 16.4 - 0.13(\text{age})$$
$$\text{SEE} = 2.5, r = -0.58, p < 0.001$$
$$\text{Sedentary subjects: METs} = 11.9 - 0.07(\text{age})$$
$$\text{SEE} = 1.8, r = -0.47, p < 0.001$$

Thus, such scales are specific to both the population tested and to whether oxygen uptake was measured directly or predicted. Note also the modest correlation coefficients ($r = -0.43$ to -0.58, a range that agrees with previous studies), which suggest that age and activity status leave a large fraction of exercise capacity unexplained. Within these limitations, equations such as these and the nomograms derived from them can provide reasonable references for normal values and can facilitate communication with patients and

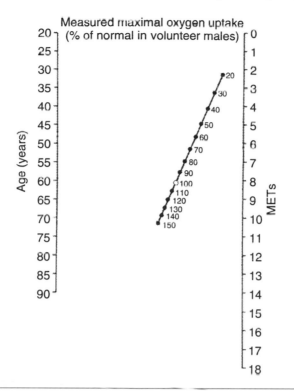

Figure 6.5 Nomogram of percent normal exercise capacity for age among 244 healthy male volunteers tested using gas exchange techniques. Reprinted from Morris et al. 1993.

between physicians regarding levels of exercise capacity in relation to their peers.

SUMMARY

This brief review of normal values suggests that a "normal" response depends greatly on the reference population and that a great deal of variability exists. The standard errors of the estimate for each regression equation suggest that 10% to 30% variation can be expected, despite extensive efforts to achieve precision by including many clinical and demographic variables. Nomograms provide an illustrative and easily applied method of estimating a normal response. The reference values described herein are not exhaustive, but represent some of the more useful or widely cited equations for gas exchange. One should consider

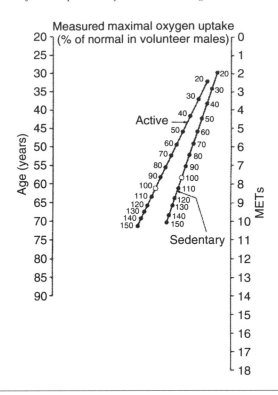

Figure 6.6 Nomogram of percent normal exercise capacity for age among active (*n* = 122) and sedentary (*n* = 74) normal male volunteers tested using gas exchange techniques. Reprinted from Morris et al. 1993.

the population being tested in one's own laboratory when choosing the most appropriate reference equations. The continued growth of gas exchange technology will undoubtedly permit more applicable, precise, and population-specific reference values.

REFERENCES

1. Jones NL. 1988. Clinical Exercise Testing, 306-311. Philadelphia: Saunders.
2. Wasserman K, Hansen JE, Sue DY, Whipp BJ. 1987. Principles of Exercise Testing and Interpretation, 72-86. Philadelphia: Lea and Febiger.
3. Hansen JE, Sue DY, Wasserman K. 1984. Predicted values for clinical exercise testing. Am Rev Respir Dis 129 (suppl): 549-555.
4. Bruce RA, Kusumi F, Hosmer D. 1973. Maximal oxygen uptake and nomographic assessment of functional aerobic impairment in cardiovascular disease. Am Heart J 85: 546-562.

5. Shephard RJ. 1969. Endurance Fitness. Toronto: University of Toronto Press.
6. Åstrand P. 1956. Human physical fitness, with special reference to sex and age. Physiol Rev 36 (suppl 2): 307-335.
7. Åstrand I. 1960. Aerobic work capacity in men and women with special reference to age. Acta Physiol Scand 49 (suppl 169): 1-92.
8. Lange-Anderson K, Shephard RJ, Denolin H. 1971. Fundamentals of Exercise Testing. Geneva: World Health Organization.
9. Morris CK, Myers J, Froelicher VF, Kawaguchi T, Ueshima K, Hideg A. 1993. Nomogram based on metabolic equivalents and age for assessing aerobic exercise capacity in men. J Am Coll Cardiol 22: 175-182.
10. Myers J, Do D, Herbert W, Ribisl P, Froelicher VF. 1994. A nomogram to predict exercise capacity from a specific activity questionnaire and clinical data. Am J Cardiol 73: 591-596.
11. Kline GM, Porcari JP, Hintermeister R, Freedson PS, Ward A, McCannon RF, Ross J, Rippe J. 1987. Estimation of $\dot{V}O_2$max from a one-mile track walk, gender, age, and body weight. Med Sci Sports Exerc 19: 253-259.
12. Froelicher VF, Thompson AJ, Noguera I, Davis G, Stewart AJ, Triebwasser JH. 1975. Prediction of maximal oxygen consumption: Comparison of the Bruce and Balke treadmill protocols. Chest 68: 331-336.
13. Milesis CA. 1993. Prediction of treadmill performance from clinical characteristics in healthy persons. J Cardiopulmonary Rehabil 7: 365-373.
14. Jackson AS, Blair SN, Mahar MT, Wier LT, Ross RM, Stuteville JE. 1990. Prediction of functional aerobic capacity without exercise testing. Med Sci Sports Exerc 22: 863-870.
15. Sue DY, Hansen JE. 1984. Normal values in adults during exercise testing. Clin Chest Med 5: 89-98.
16. Jones NL, Markrides L, Hitchcock C, Chypchar T, McCartney N. 1985. Normal standards for an incremental progressive cycle ergometer test. Am Rev Respir Dis 131: 700-708.
17. Åstrand P-O. 1952. Experimental Studies of Physical Working Capacity in Relation to Sex and Age. Copenhagen: Muskgaard.
18. Cooper CM, Weiler-Ravell D. 1984. Gas exchange response to exercise in children. Am Rev Respir Dis 129 (suppl): 547-548.

INVASIVE HEMODYNAMIC EXERCISE TESTING

*F*n certain clinical situations, more information may be needed from a patient than the standard noninvasive cardiopulmonary test offers. The term "hemodynamic testing" usually implies that central cardiac and pulmonary pressures are measured; arterial blood samples are frequently taken to calculate cardiac output, blood gases, or lactate levels. In this chapter, methods of performing this type of testing are discussed, normal hemodynamics are reviewed, and applications of hemodynamic testing in patients with cardiovascular and pulmonary disease are described.

Because these studies are invasive and require more time and skill, cost more to perform, and introduce greater discomfort and risk to the patient, they are usually reserved for patients for whom this information is likely to have a strong influence on clinical management. Flow-directed catheters can yield more precise hemodynamic information, which is sometimes useful for patients with chronic heart failure, valvular disease, and pulmonary vascular disease. For example, in addition to gas exchange data, direct information on cardiac output, filling pressure, and left ventricular end-diastolic pressure may influence treatment choices in patients with cardiomyopathy. The measurement of transvalvular gradients during exercise can greatly supplement the patient's symptoms and echocardiogram in quantifying the extent of valvular heart disease. Blood gases, including arterial PO_2, PCO_2, pH, HCO_3, and oxygen saturation obviously have a direct influence on the management of many patients with pulmonary disease and allow more direct calculations of physiologic dead space, alveolar ventilation, alveolar-arterial PO_2 difference and venous admixture.

While some centers in Europe have routinely performed either supine or upright hemodynamic studies in catheterization laboratories since the early 1970s, less has been done in the United States until recently. Much of the early information on the physiologic responses of healthy subjects to exercise and how the response of the cardiovascular system relates to performance came from hemodynamic studies performed over two decades ago (1-3). Clinically, a number of centers routinely perform these studies to help determine a patient's suitability for cardiac surgery. However, it is not at all clear that hemodynamic studies as part of the presurgical or postmyocardial infarction workup are routinely necessary. Nevertheless, in some instances the information from hemodynamic testing can significantly influence medical management. We have performed hemodynamic exercise studies only among selected patients who have been referred for coronary angiography for clinical reasons.

METHODOLOGY

Hemodynamic testing is commonly performed using a supine cycle ergometer in the catheterization laboratory. The patient's feet are attached to pedals on the ergometer, which is positioned over the catheterization table. Ergometers made for this purpose are frequently attached to the catheterization table, suspended from the ceiling, or suspended by a frame that can be wheeled into the proper position over the patient. Supine exercise can be awkward for the patient, so proper positioning of the ergometer is important. Ideally, the feet are attached securely to the pedals, the maximum flexion of the hip is 90°, and the knee reaches a near full extension with the downstroke.

Electrically braked ergometers are superior to mechanically braked ergometers for supine testing, since it is difficult to maintain the consistent revolutions per minute required for the latter, making the estimation of work difficult. The quantification of work is less of a problem when oxygen uptake is measured directly. Many catheterization laboratories are equipped with gas analysis systems that allow for the measurement of cardiac output at rest and during exercise using the Fick equation. In this setting, it is more appropriate to increment the workload moderately than outside the catheterization laboratory or when using upright exercise. Incremental stages that last 3 to 4 min usually yield steady-state conditions that can facilitate the accurate assessment of oxygen uptake, cardiac output, and pulmonary pressures. We have patients undergo exercise after baseline hemodynamic measurements are obtained. Following a return to the catheterization table (for upright studies) and a rest period, contrast angiography is then performed. Supine or upright exercise studies can be performed with catheterization by either the brachial or femoral approach. With the femoral approach, care must be taken to secure the sheaths in place and keep the manifolds and transducers stable and out of the way from leg motion.

With the patient's feet elevated above the body, intracardiac pressures increase somewhat (2 to 4 mmHg). This is due to elevation of the diaphragm and the effects of gravity, which increase venous return. Supine exercise can be awkward for the patient, and exercise capacity is considerably lower than when performed in the upright position. In addition, hemodynamic responses to exercise are markedly different. Because gravity facilitates venous return, end-diastolic volume and stroke volume are near maximal in the supine position. Thus, when comparing exercise responses in the upright and supine positions, heart rate and a-vO$_2$ difference are lower, but stroke volume and cardiac output are generally higher while supine (4,5). There is a greater total blood flow and less oxygen extraction from the blood during supine versus upright exercise. In addition, the benefits to tissue perfusion through an increase in driving force are absent in the supine position.

Upright exercise has also been performed in the catheterization laboratory, but this has been done mostly for research purposes. Upright hemodynamic testing has several advantages over supine testing. First, this position is similar to that which the patient experiences during daily activities. Pulmonary artery pressure, for example, is considerably lower in the standing versus the lying position. Efforts have been made to quantify pulmonary artery pressure changes during daily activities in patients with chronic heart failure (6). Second, for reasons mentioned earlier, the exercise response to upright exercise is far superior to that of supine exercise. Thus, if maximal hemodynamic information is important, upright exercise is a better choice. On the other hand, upright testing requires that the patient be moved from the catheterization table to the ergometer. Because the catheters must be positioned while supine, this raises obvious logistical difficulties and lessens sterility. Obtaining adequate pressure tracings during exercise can be difficult and may result in considerable artifact. We have found it useful to obtain sequential pressure recordings immediately upon ending the test with the patient sitting as motionless as possible. Most hemodynamic monitoring systems can generate mean recordings, which can be a useful supplement to the raw tracings.

Because this type of exercise testing is invasive, particular attention to patient safety is warranted. The normal contraindications to exercise apply (see Table 2.2 on p. 44). Few data are available on the risk of invasive exercise testing. Niederberger and Gaul (7) reported two cases of ventricular fibrillation and no fatalities in 8,471 tests, approximately half of which were supine and half upright.

Both cases were successfully defibrillated. It is unclear whether these incidents were caused by exercise, irritation by the catheter, or both. While these data are limited, they do suggest that the risk of complications during invasive exercise testing is similar to that reported during standard exercise testing (ranging between less than 1 to 4 per 10,000) (8,9).

As with any exercise test, the patient's symptoms, electrocardiogram, and blood pressure should be monitored continuously. Constant observation and frequent recording of hemodynamic pressures during exercise are important for safety. This permits monitoring of any fall in arterial pressure or an inordinate rise in filling pressure, and ensures that the catheters are maintained in their appropriate positions. Some patients in the catheterization setting will have disease that is too severe to exercise (such as severe heart failure, symptomatic valvular disease, or unstable angina), even though the information would appear to be useful. A catheter in the heart can induce rhythm disturbances. Exercise should be discontinued if significant symptoms occur or if hemodynamics become markedly abnormal.

APPLICATIONS OF HEMODYNAMIC EXERCISE TESTING

Some common applications of hemodynamic exercise testing include the establishment of normal hemodynamics, the determination of the degree of systolic vs. diastolic function, cardiac vs. pulmonary causes of dyspnea, and the evaluation of valvular disease. Formulas for calculating commonly measured hemodynamic variables are listed in Table 7.1.

Normal Hemodynamics

Pressure in the blood vessels created by the heart's contraction can be transmitted along a fluid-filled or transducer-tipped catheter, converted to an electrical signal, displayed on a monitor, and recorded graphically. Inflation of a balloon that occludes a segment of the pulmonary artery (''wedge'' position) permits the estimation of left atrial pressure. In most patients, the pulmonary capillary wedge pressure is an adequate reflection of left ventricular filling pressure. Two major atrial pressure waveforms, the A and the V wave, can be recorded from the right atrium and wedge positions. The A wave reflects atrial contraction. The V wave reflects venous filling of the atria during ventricular systole; the peak of the V wave occurs at the end of ventricular systole. The atrial pressure waveforms along with the ECG waveforms are commonly used as landmarks when following hemodynamic changes that occur throughout the cardiac cycle. A detailed discussion of the physiology of cardiac hemodynamics is beyond the scope of this text, but an estimation of the pressures illustrated in Figure 7.1a (p. 150) provides the

Table 7.1 Formulas for Hemodynamic Data

Variable	Calculation	Normal values at rest	Normal response to exercise
Cardiac output (L/min)	$\dfrac{\text{Oxygen uptake (ml/min)}}{\text{a-vO}_2 \text{ difference (ml O}_2/100\text{ ml)}^*}$	4-6	Up to 30
Cardiac index (CI, L/min/m²)	$\dfrac{\text{Cardiac output (L/min)}}{\text{Body surface area (m}^2)}$	2.6-4.2	Up to 20
Stroke volume (SV, ml/beat)	$\dfrac{\text{Cardiac output (ml/min)}}{\text{Heart rate (beats/min)}}$	60-100	Up to 140
Stroke volume index (SVI, ml/beat/m²)	$\dfrac{\text{Stroke volume (ml/beat)}}{\text{Body surface area (m}^2)}$	30-60	Up to 100
Stroke work (SW, g × m)	(Aortic pressure − LVEDP**) × SV × 0.0144***	60-120	Increase
Pulmonary vascular resistance (PVR, dynes × sec × cm⁻⁵)	$\dfrac{\text{Mean pulmonary arterial pressure} - \text{Mean left atrial pressure (or PCW)} \times 80}{\text{Cardiac output}}$	50-150	Decrease
Systemic vascular resistance (SVR, dynes × sec × cm⁻⁵)	$\dfrac{\text{Mean systemic arterial pressure} - \text{Mean right atrial pressure} \times 80}{\text{Cardiac output}}$	1200-1800	Decrease

*O$_2$ content for a-vO$_2$ difference calculated by % saturation × 1.36 × hemoglobin.

**LVEDP = left ventricular end-diastolic pressure.

***0.0144 is conversion factor for mmHg to cm H$_2$O.

ROUTINES TO KNOW:
A SAMPLE LABORATORY PROTOCOL

Indications for catheterization, specific equipment, procedures, and type of catheterization (right or left heart) depend on the patient and differ from laboratory to laboratory. The following is a protocol we have used when performing exercise in the catheterization laboratory. In our setting, studies are almost always restricted to right heart catheterization. This permits the acquisition of right atrial, right ventricular, pulmonary artery, and pulmonary capillary wedge pressures. In Table 7.1, computations and normal values are presented for data obtained from the combination of cardiac output by gas exchange and hemodynamic pressures.

1. Upon the patient's arrival in the laboratory, perform sterile preparation procedures.

2. Place a Swan-Ganz catheter in the usual fashion. Typically, an 8-Fr. introducer sheath is inserted into the brachial or femoral vein, and an 8-Fr. thermodilution Swan-Ganz catheter is positioned into the pulmonary artery under fluoroscopic guidance. The distal port is connected to a strain gauge transducer to permit measurements of right atrial and pulmonary artery/wedge pressures.

3. For some studies, a 5-Fr. introducer sheath is inserted into the brachial artery. This sheath is connected to a third pressure transducer for the monitoring of arterial pressure and sampling of arterial blood.

4. With the patient resting supine, begin measurements with the right atrium.

   Right Atrium (RA)

   A. Advance catheter to RA.
   B. Turn recorder on (25 mmHg scale); zero pressure.
   C. Record pressure (25 mm/sec paper speed).
   D. Record mean pressure with and without inspiration, then phasic pressure with and without inspiration.
   E. Turn recorder off.

   Right Ventricle (RV)

   A. Advance catheter to RV.
   B. Turn recorder on and record pressure (25 mm/sec paper speed).
   C. Check zero pressure.
   D. Turn recorder off.

Pulmonary Capillary Wedge (PCW)

A. Advance catheter to PCW.

B. Turn recorder on.

C. Record phasic and mean pressures (25 mm/sec paper speed).

Pulmonary Artery (PA)

A. Deflate balloon from PCW position, pull catheter back into PA position.

B. Record phasic and mean pressures (25 mm/sec paper speed).

C. Check zero pressure.

D. Turn recorder off.

E. Obtain oxygen saturation sample.

5. If supine exercise is to be performed, begin the test at this point. Obtain pressures sequentially at the end of each stage and/or as close to peak exercise as possible.

6. If upright exercise is to be performed, the sheaths are carefully secured, and the patient is helped off the catheterization table and onto a cycle ergometer placed next to the table. The patient rests 5 to 10 min while the appropriate preparations are made. These include adjusting the seat height, securing the sheaths, and carefully explaining the procedure to the patient. Obtain resting gas exchange data, zero calibrate pressures, and perform the sequence of measurements as in #4 above.

7. Begin zero-load pedaling (approximately 1 min) followed by ramp exercise (typically 10 to 15 watts/min), usually to the patient's symptom limits. Repeat the pressure measurements as close to maximum exertion as possible.

essentials for understanding basic hemodynamics during the cardiac cycle. Figure 7.1b (p. 151) illustrates normal values for oxygen saturation and oxygen content in the cardiac chambers and vessels. In Figure 7.2 (p. 152), arterial, pulmonary artery, and right atrial pressures are illustrated in a patient with coronary artery disease sitting on an upright cycle ergometer before exercising. In Figure 7.3 (p. 152), ECG and wedge pressure tracings are illustrated in a patient sitting upright at rest and at the point of maximal exertion, in which exercise is stopped and a mean recording is taken, while an effort is made to optimally position the catheter.

In earlier chapters, the direct relationship between increases in cardiac output and oxygen uptake in normal individuals was emphasized. One advantage of hemodynamic exercise testing is that cardiac output can be easily determined by directly measuring all three components of the Fick equation:

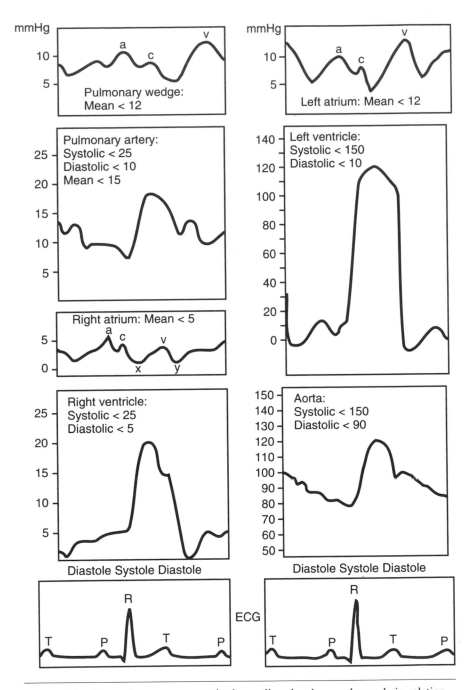

Figure 7.1a Normal pressure ranges in the cardiac chambers and vessels in relation to the ECG. Reprinted from Kern 1991.

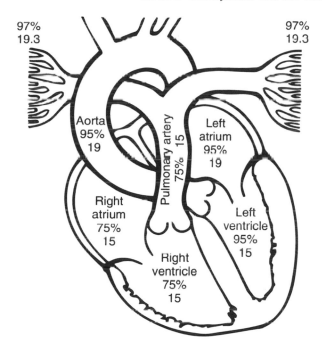

Figure 7.1b Normal values for oxygen content (volume %) and oxygen saturation (%) in the cardiac chambers and vessels. Reprinted from Kern 1991

$$\text{Cardiac output} = \frac{\text{Oxygen uptake}}{\text{a-vO}_2 \text{ difference}}$$

This is possible because a sampling port can be positioned in the pulmonary artery to obtain mixed venous blood, arterial blood can be obtained from the radial artery, and oxygen uptake can be measured with gas exchange techniques. Some laboratories calculate an ''exercise factor'' that reflects the increase in cardiac output relative to the increase in oxygen uptake during exercise. Early invasive studies suggested that cardiac output should increase approximately 600 ml for every 100 ml increase in oxygen uptake. Thus, an exercise factor less than 6.0 suggests that some pathologic process is limiting the heart's capacity to increase cardiac output in accordance with the body's demand for oxygen. To accomplish a given amount of work, these patients usually have an inordinately high oxygen extraction evidenced by a widening of the a-vO$_2$ difference.

There are several clinical situations in which invasive hemodynamic information during exercise may be indicated. These situations frequently involve patients whose clinical findings do not concur with symptoms or exercise responses. Three of the most common situations in which this can occur follow.

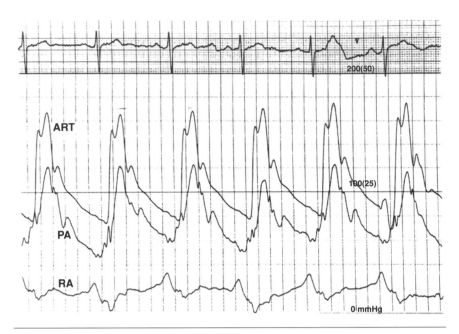

Figure 7.2 Arterial (ART), pulmonary artery (PA), and right atrial (RA) pressures in a patient sitting upright on a cycle ergometer.

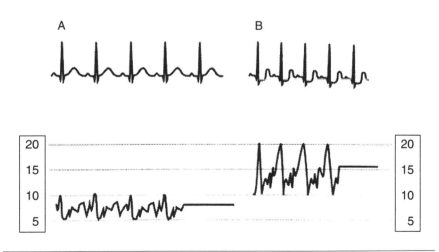

Figure 7.3 Computer-averaged waveforms of simultaneous ECG (top) and wedge pressure (bottom) recordings in a patient sitting at rest (A) and just prior to stopping at peak exercise (B). At this point exercise is stopped, and an effort is made to reposition the catheter and stabilize the recording prior to obtaining a mean value (horizontal line). Note the ST changes and the marked increase in wedge pressure from rest to peak exercise.

Systolic Versus Diastolic Dysfunction

Medical management among patients with left ventricular dysfunction has historically focused on improving systolic function. However, indices of systolic function repeatedly have been shown to be poorly related to exercise capacity (10-17). Moreover, it is well established that patients can present with classic signs and symptoms of heart failure in the presence of normal systolic function (18-21). For such reasons, diastolic function has attracted much attention in the past decade.

Several investigators have noted a close association between indices of ventricular filling and exercise tolerance, suggesting that diastolic function plays an important role in determining limitations to exercise. Diastolic dysfunction is characterized by normal cardiac output for a given workload (reflected by normal stroke volume, ejection fraction, or an exercise factor greater than 6.0), but this occurs at the expense of an elevated pulmonary wedge pressure. Left ventricular end-diastolic pressure may be normal at rest, but it will often increase in excess of 25 to 30 mmHg during exercise. Elevations in filling pressure, which are related to the dynamic compliance of the ventricle, typically reflect increases in diastolic volume. If resting compliance is poor or adapts poorly to exercise, ventricular filling is attenuated; thus, stroke volume will be reduced even in the presence of high filling pressures.

Changes in right ventricular filling pressure have been associated with improvements in submaximal exercise tolerance (22,23), and it has been suggested that patients with the most pronounced decreases in right and left ventricular filling pressures after vasodilator therapy show the largest improvements in exercise capacity and relief of symptoms (24,25). Often, minimal differences in exercise capacity are seen after therapy when no concomitant reductions in filling pressure occur. Pouleur et al. (26) studied 33 patients with mild to moderate heart failure and found that, although patients with and without reduced exercise tolerance could not be differentiated on the basis of systolic function, patients with the poorest exercise capacity had an upward shift in the diastolic pressure volume relation and higher mean ventricular filling pressures. Beta-agonist treatment with xamoterol improved exercise capacity and was accompanied by a downward shift in the diastolic pressure-volume relation.

Alternatively, poor systolic function is characterized by abnormal forward flow, causing poor stroke volume, cardiac output, ejection fraction, and an exercise factor less than 6.0. This distinction between systolic and diastolic dysfunction is an important one, as it can influence medical or even surgical management of the patient. Measures of filling pressure, ventricular compliance, and forward output require hemodynamic measurements. Obtaining some of this information during exercise can add important information regarding a patient's symptoms.

Cardiac Versus Pulmonary Dyspnea

In patients with chronic obstructive pulmonary disease, the assessment of left ventricular function can be complex (27,28). The veteran patient whom we see in our laboratory is typical in this regard, as many with left heart disease secondary to coronary artery disease, hypertension, or valvular disease have concomitant pulmonary disease. The chronic left heart diseases for which dyspnea is a hallmark have a common denominator: elevated pulmonary wedge pressure. Pulmonary wedge pressures greater than 25 mmHg are commonly observed during supine or upright exercise in patients with chronic heart failure (29-32). Despite the common association between chronic left ventricular dysfunction and elevated pulmonary wedge pressure at rest, however, note that poor relationships have been observed between pulmonary wedge pressure during exercise and exercise capacity (8,11,30,31,33,34). This observation has been used to underscore the argument that several factors are responsible for exertional dyspnea and abnormal ventilatory responses in patients with left ventricular dysfunction (see chapter 5).

Nevertheless, any elevation in pulmonary wedge pressure will increase pulmonary interstitial fluid, decrease lung compliance, and stimulate the pulmonary juxtacapillary receptors, which stimulate ventilation, leading to dyspnea. Patients with uncomplicated COPD contrast those with left ventricular dysfunction in that an elevation in pulmonary wedge pressure is unusual (35-37). In patients with COPD, pulmonary wedge pressure normally remains below 20 mmHg despite large increases in pulmonary artery pressure.

Valvular Disease

Because of reduced forward flow, aortic and mitral incompetence cause a volume overload on the left ventricle. Chronically, the left ventricle becomes enlarged. This results in predictable increases in left atrial and left ventricular filling pressures. As the left-sided pressures rise, the right-sided pressures (pulmonary arterial and pulmonary venous) must rise, too, putting added pressure on the right heart and pulmonary circulation. In patients whose valvular disease is symptomatic (causing fatigue and shortness of breath) and who are being considered for valve replacement or are undergoing angiography for the evaluation of coronary disease, it can be useful to quantify these left- and right-sided pressures during exercise to assist with decisions regarding medical or surgical management.

Like normals or other patients with heart disease, maximal oxygen uptake is limited by the patient's capacity to increase cardiac output. In mitral or aortic regurgitation, maximal cardiac output is limited by the inability of the heart to adequately increase forward flow and the extent to which chronic valvular disease has led to chronic heart failure. However, the ejection fraction may remain normal even when there is left ventricular dysfunction. It is not possible to determine from a cardiopulmonary exercise test alone whether a reduced exercise capacity in such a patient is due to chronic heart failure, valvular disease, or the degree to which the right ventricle, left ventricle, or pulmonary circulation is involved. Therefore, in some patients, hemodynamic exercise testing may be useful to elucidate more specifically the mechanism that limits the patient.

Mitral Stenosis

Mitral stenosis is defined by a reduction in the cross-sectional area of the mitral valve. Transmitral flow is dependent upon the cross-sectional area of the mitral valve, the pressure gradient between the left atrium and ventricle, and diastolic time. Mitral stenosis leads to left atrial enlargement and increases in right-sided pressures, which lead to pulmonary venous hypertension. Pulmonary vascular resistance is elevated generally in the range of 200 to 600 dynes $\times$ sec $\times$ cm^{-5}. These elevated pulmonary pressures reduce ventricular filling, resulting in reductions in cardiac output at rest and/or a failure of cardiac output to increase adequately during exercise. Hemodynamic pressures at rest and during exercise can quantify the degree to which a stenotic valve causes elevated pulmonary pressures, and they have been used to document improvements in these abnormalities and the patient's clinical status after surgery (38,39).

Aortic Stenosis

The main pathophysiologic feature of aortic stenosis is an obstruction to left ventricular outflow, resulting in a reduction in stroke volume and left ventricular dilatation. An increased left ventricular end-diastolic pressure is a hallmark of aortic stenosis, which reflects both ventricular dilatation and reduced compliance. Cardiac output is frequently normal at rest, but fails to increase appropriately with exercise. In advanced aortic stenosis, left atrial, pulmonary capillary, pulmonary arterial, right ventricular, and right atrial pressures are elevated. A large trans-valvular gradient may manifest itself during exercise and may reach a level that explains the patient's symptoms.

SUMMARY

In particular patients, a hemodynamic exercise test can help in obtaining additional diagnostic and functional information about cardiopulmonary function. These tests permit the direct measurement of central cardiac and pulmonary pressures, cardiac output, and blood gases. Because they are invasive and more costly, they are generally reserved for patients for whom the added information is likely to have a strong influence on clinical management. The few data available on risks associated with invasive hemodynamic testing do not suggest a greater complication rate than that reported for noninvasive exercise testing.

Invasive testing can be performed in either the supine or upright position, but the hemodynamic response to exercise differs considerably. In the supine position, heart rate and a-vO$_2$ difference are lower, but stroke volume and cardiac output tend to be higher during exercise when compared with the upright position. Some of the more common applications of hemodynamic exercise testing include research, the establishment of normal hemodynamics, the determination of the degree of systolic versus diastolic dysfunction, cardiac versus pulmonary causes of dyspnea, and the evaluation of valvular disease.

REFERENCES

1. Rowell LB. 1986. Human Circulation: Regulation During Physical Stress. New York: Oxford University Press.
2. Grimby G, Nilsson NJ, Saltin B. 1966. Cardiac output during submaximal and maximal exercise in active middle-aged athletes. J Appl Physiol 21: 1150-1156.
3. Vatner SF, Pagani M. 1976. Cardiovascular adjustments to exercise: Hemodynamics and mechanisms. Prog Cardiovasc Dis 19: 91-108.
4. Poliner LR, Dehmer GJ, Lewis SE, Parkey RW, Blomqvist CG, Willerson JT. 1980. Left ventricular performance in normal subjects: A comparison of the responses to exercise in the upright and supine positions. Circulation 62: 528-534.
5. Bevegard S, Holmgren A, Jonsson B. 1963. Circulatory studies in well trained athletes at rest and during heavy exercise, with special reference to stroke volume and the influence of body position. Acta Physiol Scand 57 (1-2): 26-50.
6. Gibbs JSR, Keegan J, Wright C, Fox KM, Poole-Wilson PA. 1990. Pulmonary artery pressure changes during exercise and daily activities in chronic heart failure. J Am Coll Cardiol 15: 52-61.
7. Niederberger M, Gaul G. 1983. Use of flow-directed catheters for assessment of left ventricular function during exercise: Methods, risks, and meaning for cardiac rehabilitation. J Cardiac Rehabil 3: 780-787.
8. Gibbons L, Blair SN, Kohl HW, Cooper K. 1989. The safety of maximal exercise testing. Circulation 80: 846-852.
9. Rochmis P, Blackburn H. 1971. Exercise tests: A survey of procedures, safety, and litigation experience in approximately 170,000 tests. J Am Med Assoc 217: 1061.
10. Myers J, Froelicher VF. 1991. Hemodynamic determinants of exercise capacity in chronic heart failure. Ann Intern Med 115: 377-386.
11. Szlachcic J, Massie BM, Kramer BL, Topic N, Tubau J. 1985. Correlates and prognostic implication of exercise capacity in chronic congestive heart failure. Am J Cardiol 55: 1037-1042.
12. McKirnan MD, Sullivan M, Jensen D, Froelicher VF. 1984. Treadmill performance and cardiac function in selected patients with coronary heart disease. J Am Coll Cardiol 3: 253-261.
13. Massie BM. 1988. Exercise tolerance in congestive heart failure. Role of cardiac function, peripheral blood flow, and muscle metabolism and effect of treatment. Am J Med 84: 75-82.

14. Baker JB, Wilen MM, Body CM, Dinh H, Franciosa JA. 1984. Relation of right ventricular ejection fraction to exercise capacity in chronic left ventricular failure. Am J Cardiol 54: 596-599.

15. Franciosa JA, Park M, Levine TB. 1981. Lack of correlation between exercise capacity and indexes of resting left ventricular performance in heart failure. Am J Cardiol 47: 33-39.

16. Meiler SE, Ashton JJ, Moeschberger ML, Unverferth DV, Leier CV. 1987. An analysis of the determinants of exercise performance in congestive heart failure. Am Heart J 113: 1207-1217.

17. Higginbotham MB, Morris KG, Conn EH, Coleman RE, Cobb FR. 1983. Determinants of variable exercise performance among patients with severe left ventricular dysfunction. Am J Cardiol 51: 52-60.

18. Cohn JN, Johnson G. 1990. Heart failure with normal ejection fraction. The V-Heft Study. Circulation 81 (suppl III): III-48–III-53.

19. Kessler KM. 1988. Heart failure with normal systolic function. Arch Intern Med 148: 2109-2111.

20. Dougherty AH, Maccarelli GV, Gray EL, Hicks CH, Goldstein RA. 1984. Congestive heart failure with normal systolic function. Am J Cardiol 54: 778-782.

21. Soufer R, Wohlgelernter D, Vita NA, Amuchestegui M, Sostman HD, Berger HJ, Zaret BL. 1985. Intact systolic left ventricular function in clinical congestive heart failure. Circulation 55: 1032-1036.

22. Goldsmith RL, Kukin ML, Gottlieb SS, Wilson PB, Packer M. 1988. Hemodynamic correlates of improved effort tolerance during submaximal and maximal exercise in patients with chronic heart failure (Abstract). Circulation 78 (suppl II): II-56.

23. Wilson JR, Ferraro N. 1982. Effect of isosorbide dinitrate on submaximal exercise capacity of patients with chronic left ventricular failure. Chest 82: 701-704.

24. Massie BM, Kramer B, Haughom F. 1981. Acute and long-term effects of vasodilator therapy on resting and exercise hemodynamics and exercise tolerance. Circulation 64: 1218-1226.

25. Massie BM, Kramer BL, Topic N. 1984. Lack of relationship between short-term hemodynamic effects of captopril and subsequent clinical responses. Circulation 69: 1135-1141.

26. Pouleur H, Hanet C, Rousseau MF, van Eyll C. 1990. Relation of diastolic function and exercise capacity in ischemic left ventricular dysfunction. Role of beta-agonists and beta-antagonists. Circulation 82 (2 suppl): 189-196.

27. Unger K, Shaw D, Karliner JS. 1975. Evaluation of left ventricular performance in acutely ill patients with chronic obstructive lung disease. Chest 68: 135-142.

28. Bahler RC. 1975. Editorial: Assessment of left ventricular function in chronic obstructive pulmonary disease. Chest 68: 132-133.

29. Roskamm H, Samek L, Rupp G, Schnellbacher K, Sturzenhofecker P, Petersen J, Rentrop P, Prokoph J. 1977. Can predictability of coronary

angiographic findings be improved by additional measurement of pulmonary wedge pressure during exercise? Z Kardiol 66: 477-482.

30. Sullivan MJ, Higginbotham MB, Cobb FR. 1988. Increased exercise ventilation in patients with chronic heart failure: Intact ventilatory control despite hemodynamic and pulmonary abnormalities. Circulation 77: 552-559.

31. Fink LI, Wilson JR, Ferraro N. 1986. Exercise ventilation and pulmonary artery wedge pressure in chronic stable congestive heart failure. Am J Cardiol 57: 249-253.

32. Franciosa JA, Baker BJ, Seth L. 1985. Pulmonary versus systemic hemodynamics in determining exercise capacity of patients with chronic left ventricular failure. Am Heart J 110: 807-813.

33. Lipkin DP, Canepa-Anson R, Stephens MR, Poole-Wilson PA. 1986. Factors determining symptoms in heart failure: Comparison of fast and slow exercise tests. Br Heart J 55: 439-445.

34. Wilson JR, Ferraro N. 1983. Exercise intolerance in patients with chronic left heart failure: Relation to oxygen transport and ventilatory abnormalities. Am J Cardiol 51: 1358-1363.

35. Weitzenblum E, Loiseau A, Hirth C, Mirhom R, Rasaholinjanahary J. 1979. Course of pulmonary hemodynamics in patients with chronic obstructive pulmonary disease. Chest 75: 656-662.

36. Schrijen F, Uffholtz H, Polu JM, Poincelot F. 1978. Pulmonary and systemic hemodynamics evolution in chronic bronchitis. Am Rev Respir Dis 117: 25-31.

37. Boushy SF, North LB. 1977. Hemodynamic changes in chronic obstructive pulmonary disease. Chest 72: 565-570.

38. Dalen JE, Matloff JM, Evan GL, Hoppin FG, Bhardwaj P, Harken DE, Dexter L. 1967. Early reduction of pulmonary vascular resistance after mitral-valve replacement. N Engl J Med 277: 387-394.

39. Zener JC, Hancock EW, Shumway NE, Harrison DC. 1972. Regression of extreme pulmonary hypertension after mitral valve surgery. Am J Cardiol 30: 820-826.

A

EQUATIONS FOR PREDICTING OXYGEN UPTAKE

Because the direct measurement of oxygen uptake is frequently difficult or unavailable, calculations have been standardized for predicting oxygen uptake (1). These equations should be used while keeping the caveats discussed in chapter 1 in mind. Estimated MET values are generally useful for developing an exercise prescription, using exercise capacity to determine disability, estimating prognosis, communicating with patients in terms of age-related norms, and evaluating progress.

Treadmill Walking

The equation for treadmill walking assumes that the individual is in a steady state, is not holding onto the handrails, is walking between 2 and 4 mph, and that the treadmill is calibrated. A horizontal component (speed in m/min) is added to a vertical (grade) component along with the resting metabolic rate (3.5 ml/kg/min) to yield an estimated value for oxygen uptake in ml/kg/min. Speed in mph is converted to m/min by multiplying by 26.8. For the vertical component, grade is expressed as a fraction (i.e., 5% grade equals .05).

$$\text{Horizontal component} = \text{speed (m/min)} \times 0.1 \, \frac{\text{ml } O_2/\text{kg/min}}{\text{m/min}}$$

$$\text{Vertical component} = \text{grade} \times \text{speed (m/min)} \times 1.8 \text{ ml } O_2/\text{kg/min}$$

$$\text{Resting component} = 3.5 \text{ ml } O_2/\text{kg/min}$$

For example, a person walking at 3.0 mph and 5% grade would have an estimated oxygen uptake of

---

$$\text{Horizontal component: } 3.0 \text{ mph} \times 26.8 = 80.4 \text{ m/min}$$

$$80.4 \text{ m/min} \times 0.1 \; \frac{\text{ml } O_2/\text{kg/min}}{\text{m/min}}$$

$$= 8.0 \text{ ml } O_2/\text{kg/min}$$

Vertical component: $.05 \times 80.4$ m/min $\times 1.8$ ml O_2/kg/min $= 7.2$ ml O_2/kg/min

Resting component: 3.5 ml O_2/kg/min

$$\text{Total } O_2 \text{ cost: } 8.0 \text{ ml } O_2/\text{kg/min} + 7.2 \text{ ml } O_2/\text{kg/min}$$
$$+ 3.5 \text{ ml } O_2/\text{kg/min} = 18.7 \text{ ml } O_2/\text{kg/min}$$

An alternative method that can be used is to combine the horizontal, vertical, and resting components into one equation. In the following, the units are dropped for simplicity, and, as above, grade is expressed as a fraction and mph is converted to m/min.

$$\dot{V}O_2 \text{ ml/kg/min} = \text{Speed } [0.1 + (\text{grade} \times 1.8)] + 3.5$$

For running, the oxygen cost is estimated similarly, except that speed is multiplied by a constant of 0.2 rather than 0.1 for the horizontal component, and grade is multiplied by 0.9 rather than 1.8 for the vertical component. Generally, the running equation is appropriate for speeds greater than 5.0 mph but can be used for lesser speeds as long as the individual is running.

Cycle Ergometry

Oxygen uptake is estimated on a cycle ergometer using the product of the mechanical resistance of the ergometer (in kiloponds) and the circumference of the flywheel. The "distance traveled" is equal to the number of revolutions per minute times the circumference of the flywheel. The circumference on most ergometers is either 3 or 6 m (i.e., 3 or 6 m per one revolution). Because cycle ergometry is a non-weight bearing activity, the oxygen cost is independent of body weight, and oxygen uptake is expressed in absolute terms, or milliliters per minute. Mechanical power is usually expressed in kilogram meters per minute or watts. One watt is equal to approximately 6.1 kgm/min. As with the treadmill, a resting component (3.5 ml O_2/kg/min) is added to account for the basal metabolic rate. Work on a cycle ergometer can be calculated as:

$$\dot{V}O_2 \text{ ml/min} = \text{work rate (kgm/min)} \times 2 \text{ ml/kgm}$$
$$+ \text{resting metabolic rate (ml/min)}$$

$$\text{Resting metabolic rate} = 3.5 \text{ ml } O_2/\text{kg/min} \times (\text{body weight in kg})$$

For example, for an individual who weighs 75 kg and is working at a rate of 900 kgm/min:

$$\dot{V}O_2 \text{ ml/min} = 900 \text{ kgm/min} \times 2 \text{ ml/kgm} + (3.5 \text{ ml } O_2/\text{kg/min} \times 75 \text{ kg})$$
$$= 1800 \text{ ml } O_2/\text{min} + 262 \text{ ml } O_2/\text{min}$$
$$= 2062 \text{ ml/min}$$

If the individual were performing a workload expressed in watts, the oxygen cost of the work could be estimated similarly, knowing that one watt equals roughly 6.1 kgm/min. Oxygen uptake in ml/kg/min is obtained by dividing the above value by body weight (2062 ml/min ÷ 75 kg = 27.5 ml/kg/min), and estimated METs can be obtained by dividing the ml/kg/min value by 3.5 (27.5 ÷ 3.5 = 7.5 METs).

REFERENCE

1. American College of Sports Medicine. 1995. Guidelines for Exercise Testing and Exercise Prescription, 5th ed, 269-287. Philadelphia: Lea and Febiger.

APPENDIX

B

EQUIPMENT MANUFACTURERS AND RELATED DISTRIBUTORS, ORGANIZATIONS, AND JOURNALS

Gas Exchange Equipment Manufacturers

- Medical Graphics Corporation
  350 Oak Grove Parkway
  St. Paul, MN 55127
  Telephone: (612) 484-4874
              (800) 328-4137 (Service)
              (800) 328 4138 (Sales)

- Schiller America   Main Office—Switzerland
  3002 Dow Avenue #122   Altgasse 68
  Tustin, CA 92680   CH-6340 Baar
  Telephone: (800) 247-8775   Switzerland
                                        Telephone: 042/33 43 53

- SensorMedics Corporation
  22705 Savi Ranch Parkway
  Yorba Linda, CA 92687
  Telephone: (714) 283-2228 or (800) 231-2466

- Warren E. Collins, Incorporated/Cybermedic
  220 Wood Road
  Braintree, MA 02184
  Telephone: (617) 843-0610 or (800) 225-5157

- Quinton Instrument Company
  2121 Terry Avenue
  Seattle, WA 98121-2791
  Telephone: (206) 223-7373 or (800) 426-0337

- Marquette Electronics
  8200 West Tower Avenue
  P.O. Box 23181
  Milwaukee, WI 53223
  Telephone: (414) 355-5000 or (800) 558-5120

Treadmills/Cycle Ergometers/ECG Systems

- Quinton Instrument Company
  2121 Terry Avenue
  Seattle, WA 98121-2791
  Telephone: (206) 223-7373 or (800) 426-0337

- Warren E. Collins, Incorporated
  220 Wood Road
  Braintree, MA 02184
  Telephone: (617) 843-0610 or (800) 225-5157

- Schiller America   Main Office—Switzerland
  3002 Dow Avenue #122   Altgasse 68
  Tustin, CA 92680   CH-6340 Baar
  Telephone: (800) 247-8775 Switzerland
                            Telephone: 042/33 43 53

- Marquette Electronics
  8200 West Tower Avenue
  P.O. Box 23181
  Milwaukee, WI 53223
  Telephone: (414) 355-5000 or (800) 558-5120

- Burdick Corporation
  3315 Algonquin Road
  Rolling Meadows, IL 60008
  Telephone: (800) 955-5177

- Mortara Instruments Incorporated
  7865 North 86th Street
  Milwaukee, WI 53224
  Telephone: (800) 877-8942

- Hewlett-Packard
  Diagnostic Cardiology Business Unit
  1700 South Baker Street
  McMinnville, OR 97128
  Telephone: (503) 472-5101

Face Masks, Valves, and Related Equipment

- Hans Rudolph, Incorporated
  7200 Wyandotte
  Kansas City, MO 64114
  Telephone: (816) 363-5522 or (800) 456-6695

Organizations and Related Journals

- American College of Sports Medicine
  Medicine and Science in Sports and Exercise
  P.O. Box 1440
  Indianapolis, IN 46206-1440
  Telephone: (317) 637-9200

- American Heart Association
  Circulation
  7272 Greenville Avenue
  Dallas, TX 75231-4596
  Telephone: (800) 242-8721

- American College of Cardiology
  Journal of the American College of Cardiology
  9111 Old Georgetown Road
  Bethesda, MD 20814-1699
  Telephone: (800) 253-4636

- American Association of Cardiovascular and Pulmonary Rehabilitation
  Journal of Cardiopulmonary Rehabilitation
  7611 Elmwood Avenue, Suite 201
  Middleton, WI 53562
  Telephone: (608) 831-6989

- American Physiological Society
  Journal of Applied Physiology
  9650 Rockville Pike
  Bethesda, MD 20814-3991
  Telephone: (301) 530-7160

- American Thoracic Society
  American Journal of Respiratory and Critical Care Medicine
  1740 Broadway
  New York, NY 10019-4374
  Telephone: (212) 315-6440

- American College of Chest Physicians
  Chest
  3300 Dundee Road
  Northbrook, IL 60062-2348
  Telephone: (708) 498-1400

- American Medical Society for Sports Medicine
  Clinical Journal of Sport Medicine
  7611 Elmwood Avenue, Suite 201
  Middleton, WI 53562
  Telephone: (608) 831-4484

- Canadian Academy of Sport Medicine
  R. Tait McKenzie Building
  1600 James Naismith Drive
  Gloucester, ON K1B 5N4
  Canada

LIST OF
SCIENTIFIC ABBREVIATIONS

ATge	Gas exchange anaerobic threshold
ATPS	Atmospheric temperature and pressure, saturated
a-vO₂ difference	Arteriovenous oxygen content difference
BTPS	Body temperature and pressure, saturated. Gas volume at body temperature and pressure saturated with water vapor (37 °C and 47 mmHg).
CAD	Coronary artery disease
CHF	Chronic heart failure
CI	Cardiac index, $L/min/m^2$
COPD	Chronic obstructive pulmonary disease
D	Distance
F	Force
FAI	Functional aerobic impairment
F$_E$CO$_2$	Fraction (%) of carbon dioxide in the expired air
F$_E$N$_2$	Fraction (%) of nitrogen in the expired air
F$_E$O$_2$	Fraction (%) of oxygen in the expired air
F$_{ET}$CO$_2$	Fraction (%) of end-tidal carbon dioxide
FEV$_1$	Forced expiratory volume in one second
F$_I$CO$_2$	Fraction (%) of carbon dioxide in the inspired air
F$_I$O$_2$	Fraction (%) of oxygen in the inspired air
FVC	Forced vital capacity
HCO$_3$	Bicarbonate
J	Joule
Kcal	Kilocalorie
Kgm	Kilogram × meter
Kj	Kilojoule
Kp	Kilopond
MET	Metabolic equivalent (1 MET = 3.5 ml/kg/min)
mmHg	Millimeters of mercury (pressure, tension)
MVV	Maximal voluntary ventilation, L/min

N	Newton
Nm	Newton meter
P	Power
P(A-a)O$_2$	Alveolar-arterial oxygen partial pressure difference, mmHg
P(a-ET)CO$_2$	Arterial end-tidal carbon dioxide pressure difference, mmHg
P$_a$CO$_2$	Partial pressure of carbon dioxide in arterial blood (normal is 45 mmHg)
P$_a$O$_2$	Partial pressure of arterial oxygen, mmHg
P$_A$O$_2$	Partial pressure of alveolar oxygen, mmHg
Pb	Barometric pressure, mmHg
PCO$_2$	Partial pressure of carbon dioxide, mmHg
P$_E$CO$_2$	Mixed expired carbon dioxide pressure, mmHg
P$_{ET}$CO$_2$	End-tidal carbon dioxide pressure, mmHg
P$_{ET}$O$_2$	End-tidal oxygen pressure, mmHg
pH	Hydrogen ion concentration
PO$_2$	Partial pressure of oxygen, mmHg
PTCA	Percutaneous transluminal coronary angioplasty
PVR	Pulmonary vascular resistance
Q̇	Cardiac output, L/min
RER	Respiratory exchange ratio
STPD	Standard temperature and pressure, dry. Gas volume at standard temperature (0 °C) and barometric pressure (760 mmHg), dry.
SV	Stroke volume, ml/beat
SVI	Stroke volume index, ml/beat/m^2
SVR	Systemic vascular resistance
SW	Stroke work
Ta	Ambient temperature
V̇$_A$	Alveolar ventilation, L/min
V̇CO$_2$	CO$_2$ production, L/min
V$_D$	Ventilatory dead space, ml
V$_D$/V$_T$	Ventilatory dead space to tidal volume ratio
V̇$_E$	Expired ventilation, L/min
V̇$_E$/V̇CO$_2$	Ventilatory equivalent for carbon dioxide
V̇$_E$/V̇O$_2$	Ventilatory equivalent for oxygen
V̇$_I$	Inspired ventilation, L/min
V̇O$_2$	Oxygen uptake, L/min or ml/kg/min
V$_T$	Tidal volume, ml
VT	Ventilatory threshold
W	Work

GLOSSARY

acceleration — The rate of change in velocity with respect to time.

acidosis — A high hydrogen ion concentration in the blood; pH less than 7.4.

afterload — A measure of the force resisting the ejection of blood by the heart. Determined primarily by aortic pressure.

alkalosis — A low hydrogen ion concentration in the blood; pH greater than 7.4.

alveolar ventilation ($\dot{V}_A$) — The volume of inspired air that reaches the alveoli per minute.

arteriovenous oxygen (a-vO_2) difference — The difference in oxygen content between the arterial and mixed venous blood, which reflects the amount of oxygen extracted by the tissues. Expressed in ml O_2/100 ml blood.

ATPS — An expression of gas volume under conditions of atmospheric temperature and pressure, saturated with water vapor.

Bernoulli's law — Postulate which states that the velocity of turbulent fluid movement is proportional to the square root of the change in pressure.

beta-oxidation — The initial step in fat oxidation, in which fatty acids are broken into separate 2-carbon units of acetic acid, each of which is then converted to acetyl CoA.

breathing reserve — The difference between maximal voluntary ventilation and maximal exercise ventilation.

BTPS — An expression of gas volume under conditions of body temperature and pressure, saturated with water vapor.

cardiac output ($\dot{Q}$) — The volume of blood pumped by the heart, expressed in L/min.

cardiovascular drift — Cardiovascular adjustment to prolonged exercise in which there are progressive increases in heart rate and concomitant decreases in stroke volume.

chronotropic incompetence — An abnormal heart rate response to exercise.

contractility — The force of the heart's contraction. Common measures of contractility include the ejection fraction and tension-time index.

desaturation — The unbinding of oxygen from hemoglobin.

diffusion — Passive tendency of a molecule to move from a region of higher to one of lower concentration.

dyspnea — Difficulty breathing; shortness of breath.

ejection fraction — The percentage of blood in the ventricle ejected by the heart in a single contraction. It is calculated by dividing end-systolic volume by end-diastolic volume.

emphysema — A pulmonary disease characterized by chronic obstruction, infection, and entrapment of air in the alveoli. Usually caused by long-term smoking.

end-diastolic volume — The volume of blood in the ventricle at the end of the filling phase.

end-systolic volume — The volume of blood remaining in the ventricle following the heart's contraction.

false positive response — A positive result of a diagnostic test when no disease is present.

Fick principle — Postulate which states that oxygen uptake is equal to the product of cardiac output and arteriovenous oxygen (a-vO_2) difference.

filling pressure — The pressure exerted on the heart during its diastolic phase. It is determined primarily by venous pressure.

force (F) — A basic unit of work, defined as an accelerating mass (force = mass × acceleration).

forced expiratory volume in one second (FEV_1) — The volume of air exhaled from the lungs in one second during a forceful expiration.

forced vital capacity (FVC) — The volume of air forcefully exhaled following a maximal inspiration.

Frank-Starling mechanism — The mechanism by which an increased amount of blood in the ventricle causes a more forceful contraction, increasing the volume of blood ejected.

functional aerobic impairment (FAI) — An expression of an individual's aerobic capacity (as a percentage) relative to normal for age and gender.

glycogen — Carbohydrate in its stored form in the body, primarily in the muscle and liver.

hemoglobin (Hb) — An iron-containing component of the red blood cell that binds to oxygen.

hyperventilation — Ventilation (breathing rate and/or tidal volume) beyond that required for the body's metabolic needs.

hypoxia — A reduction in the amount of oxygen.

inspired ventilation ($\dot{V}_I$) — The volume of air taken into the lungs in one minute. Conventionally expressed in L/min, ATPS.

isometric — A muscle contraction that produces no joint movement, generating force while its length remains unchanged. Also called *static*.

isotonic — A muscle contraction that produces joint movement. Also called *dynamic*.

joule (J) — A unit of work equal to one newton meter.

maximal voluntary ventilation (MVV) — The upper limit of the capacity to ventilate the lung. By convention, MVV is measured in a 12- or 15-sec interval and expressed in L/min.

metabolic equivalent (MET) — A unit used to estimate the metabolic cost of activity. One MET is equal to the approximate resting metabolic rate of 3.5 ml O_2/kg/min.

minute ventilation ($\dot{V}_E$) — The volume of air exhaled from the lungs in one minute. Conventionally expressed in L/min, BTPS.

myoglobin — A compound similar to hemoglobin, but found in the muscle tissue, which carries oxygen from the cell membrane to the mitochondria.

newton (N) — A basic unit of force, defined as the amount of force required to move a 1-kg mass 1 m × sec^{-2}.

oxygen pulse (O_2 pulse) — Oxygen uptake (ml/min) divided by heart rate (beats/min), i.e., the volume of oxygen consumed per given stroke volume.

oxygen uptake ($\dot{V}O_2$) — The common biological measure of total body work. It is defined by the rate at which oxygen is consumed by the body, expressed in L O_2/min or ml O_2/kg/min.

partial pressure — The individual pressures from each gas in a mixture.

pH — An expression of the body's hydrogen ion concentration. The normal pH of the arterial blood is 7.4.

pneumotachometer — A device that measures volume of airflow, usually by quantifying changes in pressure through a tube.

polycythemia — A condition characterized by an increase in the number of red blood cells.

power (P) — The rate at which work is performed, defined by the product of force and velocity.

preload — The force acting to stretch the myocardial fibers during diastole. Commonly estimated as left ventricular end-diastolic pressure or the end-diastolic volume.

pulmonary capillary wedge pressure — Pressure recorded with a transducer-tipped catheter when an inflated balloon occludes a segment of the pulmonary artery. In most individuals, this measurement is an acceptable reflection of left atrial pressure and left ventricular filling pressure.

respiratory exchange ratio (RER) — The ratio of expired carbon dioxide to oxygen uptake at the level of the lung.

sensitivity — A measure of the ability of a diagnostic test to correctly detect disease. Defined as the percentage of patients in whom a test gives an abnormal result when those with the disease are tested. Mathematically, sensitivity = [true positive/(true positive + false negative)].

specificity — A measure of the ability of a diagnostic test to correctly detect normals. Defined as the percentage of subjects in whom a test gives a normal result when those without disease are tested. Mathematically, specificity = [true negative/(true negative + false positive)].

steady state — A submaximal exercise condition characterized by a constant oxygen uptake.

STPD — An expression of gas volume under conditions in which temperature and pressure have been standardized (0 °C, 760 mmHg) and the gas is completely dry.

stroke volume (SV) — The volume of blood ejected per heart beat, expressed in ml/beat.

tidal volume (V_T) — The volume of air inspired or expired during a normal breathing cycle.

total peripheral resistance — The resistance of the entire systemic circulation.

true O_2 — The difference between inspired and expired oxygen content, i.e., that fraction of oxygen which has been consumed by the tissues in a given interval.

ventilation-perfusion ratio — The ratio of alveolar ventilation to alveolar capillary blood flow.

ventilatory dead space (V_D) — The volume of the respired air that does not participate in alveolar capillary gas exchange.

ventilatory threshold (VT) — The point during progressive exercise in which ventilation increases disproportionately to oxygen uptake.

ventricular compliance — The capacity of the ventricle to stretch, defined as the ratio of the change in diastolic volume to the change in transmural pressure.

V-slope — A technique for the detection of the ventilatory threshold; a nonlinear increase in CO_2 production relative to oxygen uptake.

work (W) — An expression of the force operating on a mass that causes it to change its location. Used in the context of energy expenditure, work is commonly expressed in kgm/min, J, or Kcal.

INDEX

ABOUT THE AUTHOR

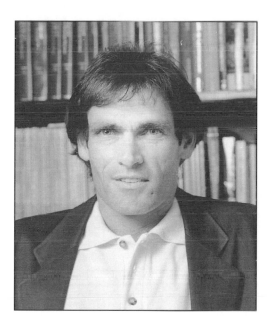

Since 1980 Jonathan N. Myers, PhD, has been researching, teaching, and writing about the significance of gas exchange techniques in cardiopulmonary exercise testing. He has conducted more than 50 workshops on the topic and consulted with manufacturers across the United States and Europe.

Publishing extensively on the topic, Myers is coauthor of the leading textbook on exercise testing, *Exercise and the Heart: Clinical Concepts*, as well as the *American Thoracic Society Standards for Clinical Exercise Testing* and the *American Heart Association Guidelines for Clinical Exercise Testing Laboratories*.

Research coordinator for the cardiology exercise laboratory at the Palo Alto VA Medical Center, Myers is also clinical assistant professor of medicine at Stanford University.

In 1991 Myers earned his PhD in exercise physiology from the University of Southern California, and in 1982 he completed his master's degree from San Diego State University. He is a member of the American College of Sports Medicine (ACSM), the American Association of Cardiovascular and Pulmonary Rehabilitation (AACVPR), and the American College of Cardiology (ACC), and he is an ACSM and ACC fellow.

Myers lives in Aptos, California, and enjoys running, basketball, and reading.

ALSO FROM HUMAN KINETICS

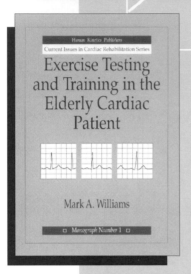

Human Kinetics Publishers
Current Issues in Cardiac Rehabilitation Series

Exercise Testing
and Training in the
Elderly Cardiac
Patient

Mark A. Williams

□ *Monograph Number 1* □

Exercise Testing and Training in the Elderly Cardiac Patient

Mark A. Williams, PhD

1994 • Paper • 136 pp
Item BWIL0621 • ISBN 0-87322-621-6
$20.00 ($29.95 Canadian)

Exercise Testing and Training in the Elderly Cardiac Patient summarizes the latest research on exercise testing and prescription for this group and provides cardiac rehabilitation specialists and students with valuable information for applying these findings in practice.

Although elderly people are the largest group of consumers of cardiac care, little study has been done on the effects of exercise testing and training on the elderly cardiac patient. In this book, groundbreaking researcher Mark Williams examines this special population and explains the art and science of tailoring programs especially for the elderly.

Working with elderly cardiac patients poses special challenges because individual ages, fitness levels, and health statuses vary so widely. Many patients also have one or more chronic diseases that affect exercise ability, including arthritis, vascular disease, and pulmonary disease. Dr. Williams describes how these factors affect exercise testing and how you can adjust your patients' exercise prescriptions accordingly.

The book's practical approach to this important topic makes it a reference you'll turn to again and again.

Prices subject to change.

Human Kinetics

The Information Leader in
Physical Activity
http://www.humankinetics.com

2335

To request information or to place your order, U.S. customers call **TOLL-FREE 1-800-747-4457**. Customers outside the U.S. use appropriate telephone number/ address shown in the front of this book.